Music Therapy and Traumatic Brain Injury

by the same author

Music Therapy and Neurological Rehabilitation
Performing Health
David Aldridge
ISBN 978 1 84310 302 8

Melody in Music Therapy
A Therapeutic Narrative Analysis
Gudrun Aldridge and David Aldridge
ISBN 978 1 85302 755 0

Music and Altered States
Consciousness, Transcendence, Therapy and Addictions
Edited by David Aldridge and Jörg Fachner
ISBN 978 1 84310 373 8

Case Study Designs in Music Therapy
David Aldridge
ISBN 978 1 84310 140 6

Music Therapy in Dementia Care
David Aldridge
ISBN 978 1 85302 776 5

Health, the Individual, and Integrated Medicine
Revisiting an Aesthetic of Health Care
David Aldridge
ISBN 978 1 84310 232 8

Spirituality, Healing and Medicine
Return to the Silence
David Aldridge
ISBN 978 1 85302 554 9

Music Therapy in Palliative Care
New Voices
David Aldridge
ISBN 978 1 85302 739 0

Music Therapy and Traumatic Brain Injury

A Light on a Dark Night

Simon Gilbertson and David Aldridge

Jessica Kingsley Publishers
London and Philadelphia

First published in 2008
by Jessica Kingsley Publishers
116 Pentonville Road
London N1 9JB, UK
and
400 Market Street, Suite 400
Philadelphia, PA 19106, USA

www.jkp.com

Library of Congress Cataloging in Publication Data
Gilbertson, Simon.
  Music therapy and traumatic brain injury : a light on a dark night / Simon Gilbertson and
David Aldridge.
     p. ; cm.
  Includes bibliographical references.
  ISBN 978-1-84310-665-4 (pb : alk. paper) 1. Brain damage--Patients--Rehabilita-
tion--Case studies. 2. Music therapy--Case studies. I. Aldridge, David, 1947- II. Title.
     [DNLM: 1. Brain Injuries--rehabilitation--Case Reports. 2. Music
Therapy--methods--Case Reports. WL 354 G466m 2008]
     RC387.5.G525 2008
     616.89'1654--dc22
                                                        2008004133

British Library Cataloguing in Publication Data
A CIP catalogue record for this book is available from the British Library

ISBN 978 1 84310 665 4

This book is dedicated to Keith Gilbertson

Acknowledgements

In 1994, as the clinical work, which is the heart of this book, began at Klinik Holthausen in Hattingen, Germany, there were no textbooks or guidelines on music therapy in rehabilitation and traumatic brain injury.

We therefore gratefully acknowledge and honour the individuals and families affected by traumatic brain injuries with whom we have experienced the process of rehabilitation.

Our thanks go to Professor Werner Ischebeck and all our colleagues at the Klinik Holthausen for their support. In particular, we would like to thank Christian Sievert, the financial director, and Dr Michael Amend, the acting medical director, for their friendship and continuous support to Simon and the large team of music therapists who have worked at the clinic. We are also grateful to the worldwide group of music therapists in neurorehabilitation for their experience and collaboration.

We would like to thank our colleagues and the doctoral candidates at the Chair of Qualitative Research in Medicine, Institute of Music Therapy, University of Witten, Germany who supported Simon during his doctoral research which is reported in this book. Our particular thanks go to our colleague and great friend, Professor Lutz Neugebauer, the leader of the Institute for many years, who has co-founded the Nordoff-Robbins Centre, Witten, Germany with David.

We would also like to thank Professor Mícheál Ó Súilleabháin, the director of the Irish World Academy of Music and Dance, and Professor Jane Edwards, the course director of the MA in Music Therapy, for creating the opportunity for Simon to join them in developing music therapy through the Irish World Academy of Music and Dance, University of Limerick, Ireland.

Finally, David would like to thank Gudrun and Simon would like to thank Joy and Tanja, Ben and Tom, for their love and inspiration.

Contents

List of Tables

List of Figures

CHAPTER 1

Traumatic Brain Injury and Rehabilitation

The room is cool and silent. The elusive smell of disinfection fluid and rosemary tells the tale of the early morning rounds by nurses and auxiliaries. A young man lies in one of the two hospital beds, his head turned away from the therapist. His face extends beyond the white and yellow striped sheets. The therapist notes:

> As I walk towards him, he doesn't turn towards me. At his bedside, I see he is looking in my direction but I am not sure if we are sharing eye contact. I express my hope that I am not intruding after entering the room uninvited and explain who I am and why I am here. During these few moments, it is clear that he cannot speak, nor does he make any vocal sounds. Apart from his chest rising and falling, Mark does not move and remains silent.

It was only a few days since he lost control of his motorcycle on a quiet countryside road during a ride in the sunshine. A previously young and active man, now rendered immobile and damaged.

About this book

For people who have experienced traumatic brain injury, meaning and sense in life may become disrupted, distorted and, for some, hidden. The effects of traumatic brain injury are disastrous and the sudden and extreme nature of physical and psychological insult is unimaginable. Each individual who has experienced traumatic brain injury will require individual attention and express personal needs and wishes throughout his or her path of rehabilitation. A central question that will be discussed in this book is 'How can music in therapy be used to attend to the personal needs and wishes of a person who has experienced traumatic brain injury?' A particular emphasis will be made on the improvisational aspects of music as related to what the patient does. This has been emphasized as the performative aspect of music therapy and becoming a person (Aldridge 1995, 2005).

At the time when the case material for this book was being collected, clinics for the early rehabilitation of patients following neurosurgery were novel. Only a handful of such rehabilitation clinics existed throughout Germany. Since the early 1990s there has been a significant expansion of the clinical application of music therapy in the area of neurorehabilitation. Medical journals have been prepared to publish this work, recognizing its significance for rehabilitation in terms of a non-technological intervention that emphasizes human relationship and contact (Aldridge, Gustorff & Hannich 1990). Worldwide, music therapists have begun turning their attention to the possibilities music therapy can provide in this setting. We saw in previous books how music therapy is emerging as an effective intervention in the field of neurological rehabilitation (Aldridge 2005) and how case study designs are an important form of documentation (Aldridge 2004a). In this book we take these initial discussions one step further.

In music therapy sessions with people who have experienced traumatic brain injury, people who have initially been labelled as 'non-reacting' or 'unreachable' have begun to sing and play musical instruments. Single, breathy, vocal utterances have completed cadences and led to a sharing of melodic phrases. Finger movements limited by spastic muscle patterns and so fine that they must be described in millimetres have determined the direction of musical improvisations and dialogues. These fine, often minute, movements and vocal sounds have sometimes developed into a repertoire of physical and communicative gestures that can form the basis of developing relationships in the context of shared musical activities. Gigantic, explosive explorations of steel drums, gongs and large drums have contrasted the stillness of patients no longer able to speak.

As one of the intervention forms in music therapy, music improvisation has shown great potential to be a significant activity in rehabilitation processes for some people who have experienced traumatic brain injury.

Changes in health care provision are leading to a reduction of services. In times when leaders of health care services are challenged to achieve a healthy budget, decisions about the best possible health care provision may be compromised. These decisions may be supported if clear evidence of effectiveness can be consulted. Often, discussions about the necessity of music therapy in neurosurgical rehabilitation have been hampered by the absence of any 'accepted' evidence of effectiveness. Without this resource, the discussions have been reduced to a consideration of whether the music therapy is affordable.

Music therapists working in neurorehabilitation have focused both on functional and psychological issues. As Wit and colleagues (1994) have written:

> the history of music therapy suggests that cognitive issues have always been a part of the scope of the field when working with the neurologically impaired. If music therapy intervention is to be 'holistic', then cognitive needs must be addressed when working with brain-injured individuals in music therapy, though not to the exclusion of emotional, psychosocial, and physical needs. (p.86)

Music therapy *researchers* have however not focused on these aspects of clinical practice and have, with the exclusion of one study (Magee & Davidson 2002), focused on functional aspects of neurorehabilitation.

Is it the difficulty in showing change in emotional process that turns clinicians and researchers to focus upon functional ability? Standard methods in controlled quantitative research may not be capable of measuring change in some of the non-standardized qualities of human life. People who have experienced traumatic brain injury may experience loss of functional, emotional, social and cultural existence. The decision of a profession to focus on any one of these facets may be made on the evidence of potential gain for the recipients of the therapeutic intervention. In 1999 the music therapist Wendy Magee wrote:

the social and emotional needs of the client are often seen as being less important than the more visible functional needs and certainly appear more difficult to measure objectively...it is often immensely difficult to illustrate the value of this type of contact in a neuro-rehabilitation setting in any quantifiable way, other than incorporating more physical and functional goals within a music therapy program. In doing so, however, we risk neglecting the enormous potential for emotional rehabilitation which music therapy offers. (p.20)

We have consistently emphasized the holistic importance of music interventions encouraging the integrative aspects of music therapy in medical settings, particularly as such an approach does not shy away from neither the psychosocial nor the emotional as they inevitably occur in a culture of healing intentions (Aldridge 2004b).

Traumatic brain injury

Definition

Traumatic brain injury is a form of acquired brain damage and is defined as 'damage to living brain tissue caused by an external, mechanical force' (Lemkuhl 1992).

In their discussion of traumatic brain injury, also known as craniocerebral trauma, Adams and Victor (1989) say that

the basic process is at once both simple and complex – simple because there is usually no problem about etiologic diagnosis, viz., a blow to the head – and complex because of uncertainty about the pathogenesis of the immediate cerebral disorder and a number of delayed effects that may complicate the injury. (p.693)

In 1986 the National Head Injury Foundation published the following definition of traumatic head injury:

Traumatic head injury is an insult to the brain, not of a degenerative or congenital nature but caused by an external physical force, that may produce a diminished or altered state of consciousness, which results in impairment of cognitive abilities or physical functioning. It can also result in the disturbance of behavioural or emotional functioning. These may be either temporary or permanent and cause partial or total functional disability or psychological maladjustment. (in Synder Smith & Winkler 1990, p.347)

Van Dellen and Becker (1991) describe the two major forms of damage involved in a craniocerebral trauma. Injury occurring at time of trauma 'produces *primary* damage to a highly integrated system that is almost entirely lacking the ability for functional repair' (p.861). At any time following this initial event 'the damaged neural tissue is extremely vulnerable to additional *secondary* insults. The processes then initiated, which are often dynamic, can produce further permanent damage or compromise marginal structures and functions' (ibid.).

Sequelae of traumatic brain injury

The diagnosis of the sequelae of traumatic brain injury (TBI) occurs over a span of time. Directly after traumatic brain injury 'the immediate clinical aspects of traumatic head injury can include alterations in autonomic function, consciousness, motor function, pupillary responses, ocular movement and other brain stem reflexes' (Synder Smith & Winkler 1990, p.349). Autonomic functions are regulatory mechanisms controlling pulse, respiration, temperature, blood pressure, sweating and salivation.

The most common sequelae of TBI include changes in consciousness, motor disturbances, memory impairments, speech/language disorders, disorders of cognition, behavioural changes and disorders of bodily functions. The consequences of TBI can be understood along 'a continuum from altered physiological functions of cells through neurological and psychological impairments, to medical problems and disabilities that affect the individual with TBI, as well as the family, friends, community, and society in general' (National Institute of Health (NIH) Consensus Development Panel on Rehabilitation of Persons with Traumatic Brain Injury 1999, p.976).

Traumatic brain injury is caused by an event of traumatic and dramatic nature. This event can lead to complex and life-threatening challenges to the patient. These injuries, often occurring within seconds or less, may affect the whole remaining life of the person and, 'in many cases, the consequences of TBI endure in original or altered forms across the lifespan, with new problems likely to occur as the result of new challenges and the aging process' (NIH Consensus Development Panel on Rehabilitation of Persons with Traumatic Brain Injury 1999, p.976).

Epidemiology of head injury

To gain a wider perspective upon the significance of head injury we will need to assess the risk of sustaining a head injury for each 'healthy' person or member of a defined population. There is no standardized global definition of head injury, and there is no consensus in the literature about the specific definition of the term 'traumatic brain injury'. For these reasons it is only possible to report the individual epidemiological data of related studies. A single statement about the epidemiology of traumatic brain injury is not possible. The collection of data about the epidemiology of traumatic brain injury is also complicated by the lack of centralized registration of injuries and not all people experiencing traumatic brain injury are registered. In addition, people who have experienced very mild traumatic brain injury may not present to hospital at all.

The European Brain Injury Consortium Survey of Head Injuries

The European Brain Injury Consortium (EBIC) surveyed contemporary practice in the treatment of head injured individuals in 1995 (Murray *et al.* 1999). Sixty-seven neuro centres based in 12 European countries took part in the study. The 1005 patients involved in this study were assessed on the Glasgow Coma Scale as clinically presenting either 'severe' or 'moderate' coma.

An analysis of the causes of injuries shows both unintentional and intentional injuries. Road-traffic accidents (RTAs) are responsible for 52% of all injuries alongside injuries related to work, assault, domestic incidents, sport, falls under the influence of alchol and others (Murray *et al.* 1999).

Road-traffic accidents are responsible for a large number of the most severe and fatal injuries to individuals injured in many European and non-European countries. Males are significantly more at risk of being killed or injured as result of a traffic accident than females. The occupants of vehicles are at the highest risk of being severely or fatally injured in a traffic accident in comparison to all other types of transport.

Injury caused by road-traffic accidents

As the aforementioned study shows, road-traffic accidents are the most common cause for traumatic brain injury. People suffering traumatic brain injury in road-traffic accidents are most likely to suffer severe or most severe brain injuries. As an indicator of the size of impact upon the global community, statistics concerning injury related to road-traffic accidents are of interest.

Injury caused by road-traffic accidents was estimated as the ninth highest cause for life years spent with disability in 2002 (World Health Organization 2004). Globally, road-traffic injuries were the sixth most common cause of Disability Adjusted Life Years (DALYs) for males and the fifteenth most common cause of DALYs for females (World Health Organization 2004).

Epidemiology of head injury caused by road-traffic accidents in the future

In 1997 the Global Burden of Disease Study created three alternative projections for changes in the causes of death and disability (Murray & Lopez 1997). The three epidemiological profiles calculated baseline, optimistic and pessimistic estimations for the causes of death and disability in the year 2020. The projection for the number of deaths and DALYs caused by road-traffic accidents is of interest here. By 2020 road-traffic accidents have been projected in the baseline profile to move up six positions in the ranking to become the third most common cause of death. Road-traffic accidents are also projected to become worldwide the third largest cause for DALYs in 2020 and are also expected to increase by 107.6%.

Significant differences are seen when epidemiological data for developed and developing regions is compared. Road-traffic accidents are projected to become the fourth most common cause of disability in the developed regions and will be responsible for 6.9 million DALYs or 4.3% of all causes. In developing regions road-traffic accidents are projected to become the second most common cause of disability in 2020 and be the cause of 64.4 million DALYs or 5.24% of all causes.

Road-traffic accidents are estimated as being responsible for 37.7 million DALYs for the year 2001. This makes up 2.6% of all causes of disability. Males were significantly more at risk from road-traffic accidents (3.4%) than females (1.6%) at a global level (World Health Organization 2002).

Projections made by the Global Burden of Disease Study in 1997 (Murray & Lopez 1997) show a significant increase in the number of individuals injured by traffic accidents. We will be able to see whether the magnitude of the projections for 2020 becomes reality in future years. What seems to be certain is that the number of individuals requiring care and support after surviving severe road-traffic accidents will increase.

Rehabilitation

The term 'rehabilitation' is used in two ways. First, to describe health care treatments provided. Second, to determine specific phases in health care treatment systems.

Rehabilitation as a form of health care treatment

The word 'rehabilitation' derives from the Latin term *rehabilitare*, meaning 'to restore to a previous condition; to set up again in proper condition' (Friedrichsen 1980). Another definition is 'restore to health or normal life by training and therapy after imprisonment, addiction, or illness' (Soanes & Stevenson 2003). These definitions emphasize an expectation of rehabilitation to return an individual to a previous, earlier and normal state. In neurosurgical rehabilitation it is misleading to consider rehabilitation only from this restorative perspective. As a result of traumatic brain injury, people change. Many patients following illness or disease requiring neurosurgical attention have experienced such change that it is inappropriate to consider these in simple terms of reversibility. Definitions of contemporary neurorehabilitation emphasize the need for co-active involvement of the patient and therapist in a process of adaptation to life possibly with disabilities.

The World Health Organization defined the term 'rehabilitation' as 'the combined and coordinated use of medical, social, educational and vocational measures for training or retraining the individual to the highest possible level of functional ability' (World Health Organization 1969, cited in Glanville 1982, p.7).

The English neurorehabilitation specialist Barbara Wilson describes rehabilitation as a 'two way process'. She states:

> Unlike treatment, which is given *to* a patient, rehabilitation is a process in which the patient, client or disabled person takes an active part. Professional staff work together with the disabled person to achieve the optimum level of physical, social, psychological, and vocational functioning. The ultimate goal of rehabilitation is to enable the person with a disability to function as adequately as possible in his or her most appropriate environment. (1999, p.13)

From this description, we can understand rehabilitation as a collection of activities that rely on the recognition of the patient's needs, wishes and environmental context.

Rehabilitation is also a return to former habits and to the patient's own place in an ecological niche. To achieve a positive rehabilitation we may have to consider working with the ecological niche, that is those persons in the relational and environmental environment of the patient, as well as with the person alone. What identity we achieve in the future is dependent upon our own activities and what others allow us to have. We saw in our work with multiple sclerosis patients that achieving an identity as an active creative person played an important role in being healthy in daily life (Aldridge 2005; Schmid & Aldridge 2004).

The National Institute of Health Consensus Development Panel on Rehabilitation of Persons with Traumatic Brain Injury (1999) published the results of a conference in which reviews of expert opinion and a comprehensive literature review were used 'to provide biomedical researchers and clinicians with information regarding and recommendations for effective rehabilitation measures for persons who have experienced a traumatic brain injury' (p.974). In this report, the NIH Development Panel state that 'the goals of cognitive and behavioral rehabilitation are to enhance the person's capacity to process and interpret information and to improve the person's ability to function in all aspects of family and community life' (p.978). Two forms of activities have been identified in this review, restorative and compensatory approaches: 'restorative training focuses on improving a specific cognitive function, whereas compensatory training focuses on adapting to the presence of a cognitive deficit' (ibid.). The modalities of therapies described in this report include cognitive exercises, psychotherapy, pharmacological agents, behaviour modification, vocational rehabilitation and comprehensive interdisciplinary rehabilitation. The NIH Development Panel refer to music therapy, saying 'other therapies, such as structured adult education, nutritional support, art and music therapy, therapeutic recreation, acupuncture, and other alternative approaches, are used to treat persons with TBI. These methods are commonly used, but their efficacy has not been studied' (p.979).

The NIH Development Panel (1999, p.980) recommend:

- Rehabilitation services should be matched to the needs, strengths, and capacities of each person with TBI and modified as those needs change over time.

- Rehabilitation programmes for persons with moderate or severe TBI should be interdisciplinary and comprehensive.

- Rehabilitation of persons with TBI should include cognitive and behavioural assessment and intervention.

Welter and Schönle (1997, p.2) refer to four central concerns expressed by the World Health Organization about rehabilitation:

- Rehabilitation, as a rule, does not lead to profit.

- The aims of rehabilitation should not be oriented to economical factors.

- Rehabilitation is a social strategy, that aims at a fair and equal society.

- Rehabilitation is a measure of our willingness to cooperate with the poorest, the most dependent and the under-privileged in our society.

As we see, rehabilitation is understood as a necessary element of our society that is based on participation and equality, regardless of health situation. As Aldridge (2001, p. 1) remarks, 'We are challenged as a society that people within our midst are suffering and it is our responsibility within the delivery of health care to meet that challenge with appropriate responses.'

Phases of rehabilitation

To differentiate between the necessary resources for the treatment of severely injured individuals, definitions for differing phases of treatment have been implemented.[1] The definition of these phases is not based on the time point of treatment but on the severity of the disability. Following the suggestions of Welter and Schönle (1997) the following 'Phase Model' has been adopted:

Phase A   Acute treatment

Phase B   Early rehabilitation

Phase C   Continuing rehabilitation

Phase D   General rehabilitation, follow-up rehabilitation

In this book we focus on rehabilitation in Phases B and C. Admission and discharge from these phases are determined by the severity of illness and accompanying symptoms. Phase B relates to the process of rehabilitation during which there is no current indication for neurosurgical treatment such as intracranial pressure or sepsis, and the patient must breathe without mechanical assistance (von Wedel-Parlow & Kutzner 1999). In this phase the patient is commonly incontinent, fed artificially via a feeding tube and requires total assistance from nursing staff (von Wedel-Parlow & Kutzner 1999). The shift to Phase C rehabilitation is considered when the patient is able to be partially mobilized in a wheelchair for short periods, may demonstrate some participation and co-operation, and requires less than 4–5 hours of nursing care per day (von Wedel-Parlow & Kutzner 1999).

1   These phases follow the guidelines of the Bundesarbeitsgemeinschaft für Rehabilitation (BAR) and the Arbeitsgruppe Neurologie des Verbands deutscher Rentenversicherungsträger (VDR).

CHAPTER 2

Music Therapy with People Who Have Experienced Traumatic Brain Injury: What the Literature Says

For many patients the initial weeks following severe traumatic brain injury are characterized by a loss of usual interaction with the environment. When closely observed the individuals may seem completely absent of movement or vocalizations. In some instances families and caretakers may occasionally observe minimal and undirected physical movements or vocal utterances.

Music therapists initially approach these individuals from a 'listening perspective' and concentrate on any sounds or movements the patients may make. This observational perspective provides a sensitive basis for assessing any actions made by the patient within the context of the presented music therapy intervention and, it is argued, a unique form of diagnostic potential (Bischof 2001; Gadomski & Jochims 1986; Gilbertson 1999; Herkenrath 2002; Jones 1990; Noda *et al.* 2003; Tamplin 2000; Tucek, Auer-Pekarsky & Stepansky 2001).

Gadomski and Jochims (1986) suggest through observation and interpretation of the patient's musical actions and non-musical behaviour during interactive music improvisation that it may be possible to gain unique information about the condition of the patient in terms of awareness, perception of the environment and communicative ability.

This source of information may provide additional insight into the condition of patients who show minimal or no observable responses in usual diagnostic situations.

Tamplin (2000) describes observing positive changes in breathing, eye movement and eye contact of four adults whilst improvising vocally. The synchronization of breathing tempo and music tempo and changes in eye activity are interpreted as signs of the patient's awareness of the music and the music therapist. Changes in tension and relaxation are regarded as indicators of the patient's music perception and listening.

Improvised music offers a strategy of evaluating the perception and orientation of patients with severe brain injury who present either minimal or no observable actions or reactions (Herkenrath 2002). Herkenrath suggests that a range of observable qualities including breathing, mimic, body movement and vocalizations can provide a basis and content for music improvisation. This form of intervention aims to assist the patient in regaining orientation to their body, space, time, place and intentionality of action.

In 1990 Jones published a report of a young male patient for whom pre-recorded music was played via headphones following the initiative of his primary nurse. The patient had experienced traumatic head injury and was considered not to be able to respond. A cassette recording of music, heard by the patient and his wife before the accident, started a chain of events that demanded the primary nurse to re-evaluate the diagnosis of persisting vegetative state. The nurse reports how the patient suddenly began to cry. As the nurse turned the music off the patient's 'eyes became dark and he shook his head vigorously, dislodging the headphones' (Jones 1990, p.196). As the nurse asked whether he wanted to continue listening to the music, the patient responded with slow and deliberate nodding. After recognizing the patient's ability to respond, the nurse encouraged and supported the patient in developing a wider range of communication. The patient increased shaking his head and added shrugging his shoulders to answer questions with gestures. Though this report does not represent the work of a music therapist, it does emphasize the potential music may hold for some patients with traumatic brain injuries to enter into a dialogue with their environment. More recently, Noda and colleagues (2003) also emphasized the significance of careful visual and aural observation of patients following severe traumatic brain injury.

Observable changes in the awareness of the immediate environment are clinically highly significant in the early phases of rehabilitation following traumatic brain injury. These signs may include changes in breathing, vocalizations or minute body movements.

Two children (aged seven and ten) received music therapy as a part of their rehabilitation following severe injuries as passengers in a motor vehicle accident (Kennelly and Edwards 1997). Improvised singing was used to encourage potential communicative actions during coma and coma emergence. In improvisation the therapist musically mirrored the non-musical actions of the children, such as minimal body movement. During the therapy process, both children presented patterns of eye opening and attempts to speak which were understood as 'behaviours indicative of improvements in orientation and awareness' (ibid., pp.23–4).

> It may be said that breath is the chain that links body, heart and soul together, and is so important that the body – so loved and cared for, kept in palaces, its slightest cold or cough treated by doctors and medicines – is of no more use and cannot be kept anymore when the breath is gone. (Khan 1991, p.71)

Aldridge has constantly emphasized the integrative aspects of breath and that mastery of the breath is vital (Aldridge 1989, 2002, 2004b). It is the intention of the healer, reaching out with his or her own breath, to balance the breath of the patient through rhythm. Through this intended breath we see an improvement in consciousness. Breathing is a central principle in communication and healing, and forms the basis of so many therapeutic disciplines that we would perhaps be advised to encourage our clinicians towards their breath and away from their machines. Indeed, working at the Memorial Sloan-Kettering Cancer Center in New York, the intensive care medical team emphasize this personal, relational, non-technological approach as a balance to the necessary high-tech interventions. (Note that we are emphasizing a complementary balancing intervention, not an alternative.)

On this basis, singing is a logical and essential consequence for a healing initiative.

Awareness, orientation and memory

Improvised songs have been used in therapy with people who have experienced traumatic brain injuries. This technique has been used to increase the patient's environmental awareness by relating the song text to the actual activities (Claeys *et al.* 1989). Improvised song has been also used as a part of reality orientation therapy in which text related to the weather, the date and time of day has been incorporated (ibid.). Baker (2001) also highlights the importance of music therapy techniques that lead to statistically significant positive changes in the orientation of patients who have suffered post-traumatic amnesia and shows that playing live or recorded music leads to an increase in orientation and memory.

Baker (2001) also shows that people experiencing post-traumatic amnesia recall events that occur in the music therapy intervention better than events occurring in other situations. This provides strong support for the provision of music therapy at early stages of rehabilitation of people with post-traumatic amnesia. Jochims (1990) reports a patient with transitional psychosis who was able to remember a greeting song used in the music therapy setting from the phase of treatment otherwise forgotten.

Knox and Jutai (1996) suggest music listening activities are effective in music-based attention rehabilitation because specific neural pathways are activated: 'The partial localization of attention and musical processing in the right temporo-parietal lobe areas suggest that music seems to engage the most important and complex neural system for human attention and memory' (p.74). Wit *et al.* (1994) carried out an investigation into the effects of electro-acoustic music-based attention training with adolescents who had suffered closed head injuries. Though inconclusive, the results suggest further enquiry is warranted into the potential of this method in facilitating positive improvement in sustained and alternating/divided attention.

Speech and language

Many authors refer to the benefits of music therapy strategies in the rehabilitation of speech and language disorders resulting from traumatic brain injury (Aldridge 1993; Baker and Wigram 2004; Bischof 2001; Cohen 1992; Emich 1980; Jungblut 2003; Kennelly, Hamilton & Cross 2001; Livingston 1996; Lucia 1987; Magee 1999; Robb 1996).

Alongside vocal exercises, pre-composed song and song creation, improvised singing has been used in joint music and speech therapy interventions with children who have experienced TBI (Kennelly *et al.* 2001). Combinations of music therapy techniques (in Kennelly & Edwards 1997) were used with children emerging from coma and post-coma. Joint therapy approaches join elements of music and speech therapy interventions to meet the specific needs of children with speech/language dysfunction following TBI.

Emotional expression

Music therapy has been suggested as a relevant therapeutic strategy in providing patients with traumatic brain injury with an adequate form of emotional expression (Bright & Signorelli 1999; Burke *et al.* 2000; Gadomski and Jochims 1986; Gilbertson 1999; Glassman 1991; Hiller 1989; Jochims 1990, 1992; Robb 1996).

Notable changes are observed in the areas of enjoyment, sense of individuality and the ability to express emotion measured in the authors' own Quality of Life assessments during the individual music therapy sessions (Bright & Signorelli 1999).

Change in mood

Nayak and colleagues (2000) identified changes in their study of the effects of group music therapy with 18 hospitalized patients following stroke or traumatic brain injury. The music therapy interventions used were 'typical of music therapy practice' (p.278) and included a welcome song or activity, followed by instrumental improvisation, singing, composition, playing instruments, performing or listening to music. Positive trends were seen in mood state in a week-to-week comparison made by family members ($p<0.6$). Weak positive trends were observed in the measurement of mood in self-report ($p<0.10$) and family rating in a day-to-day comparison ($p<0.10$). Baker (2001) also identified statistically significant positive change in the reduction of agitation in a group of patients suffering from post-traumatic amnesia ($p<0.0001$). No statistical difference was observed between the effects of the live or recorded presentation of the music intervention.

Level of involvement in rehabilitation

One of the difficulties of rehabilitation is motivating the person who has been injured to take an active part in the rehabilitation process. Recovery means performing, and being severely injured often means that getting engaged in activities is extremely challenging and confronting.

Barker and Brunk (1991) describe the role of music improvisation in the context of a Creative Arts Therapy Group to increase active participation and a commitment to group attendance.

In 1994 Jochims described how a musically experienced patient with disturbed musical ability, as a result of traumatic brain injury, regained the ability to play music in a structured and rhythmically organized manner through music improvisation techniques (Jochims 1994). The author describes the patient as being more active and involved in music therapy than in all other situations in the rehabilitation clinic. This contrast is related to the fact that his 'inner drive was missing to confront the uncomfortable elements of daily life' (ibid., p.1323). This implies that music therapy can offer patients the opportunity to behave differently in music therapy sessions compared to other situations and settings.

Interpersonal aspects of human experience are commonly neglected in neurorehabilitation

Jochims (1992) suggests that basic functional ability is a prerequisite for self-dependency, a reduction in required assistance in self-care and increased participation in everyday life. However, he argues that intra- and interpersonal aspects of human experience are commonly neglected in neurorehabilitation. By attending to the emotional and psychological state of these patients, music improvisation in therapy can provide a balance for the dominating aspect of functional retraining of physical ability. In this sense music therapy provides a balance to the overall rehabilitative treatment strategy.

Magee (1999, p.20) stresses:

> the social and emotional needs of the client are often seen as being less important than the more visible functional needs and certainly appear more difficult to measure objectively...it is often immensely difficult to illustrate the value of this type of contact in a neuro-rehabilitation setting in any quantifiable way, other than incorporating more physical and functional goals within a music therapy program. In doing so, however, we risk neglecting the enormous potential for emotional rehabilitation which music therapy offers.

Magee points here to an important issue for researchers in the field of neurorehabilitation. It is obvious in the identified literature that researchers are aware of difficulties when challenged to demonstrate effectiveness of music therapy as a significant therapeutic strategy in emotional rehabilitation. Do difficulties in the use of research methods turn clinicians and researchers to focus on functional ability and to move away from central facets of clinical music therapy? Research pertains to the development of clinical practice and not to the disintegration of clinically relevant intervention strategies. Standard methods in controlled quantitative research may simply not be capable of measuring change in some of the non-standardized qualities of human life. Music therapy researchers in neurorehabilitation are not challenged to create a new and complex solution to this dilemma, but should look towards becoming proficient in research methods that actually fit clinically relevant questions (Aldridge 2001, 2004b). How can researchers be expected to provide evidence of effectiveness if their own work is hindered by methodological inappropriateness? Because of this, clinicians and researchers are recommended to look towards strategies of clinical research such as case study methods (Aldridge 2004a) that stay close to practice.

Independence

Following traumatic brain injury, many individuals experience changes in their functional independence, for instance in terms of getting dressed (Gervin 1991) and safe wheelchair use (Lee & Baker 1997).

Independency consists of many areas of agency and is defined by each individual. For people who have experienced TBI, basic abilities such as eating and drinking may be primary issues in regaining initial independence (Yamamoto *et al.* 2003).

Identity

We have suggested earlier that achieving a new identity is a central feature of neurological rehabilitation. Do we see ourselves as damaged and disabled or as persons made new? This is a central existential question of recovery for many people who have been ill (Aldridge 1996, 2000, 2005).

Music improvisation has been used successfully in therapy to assist the redevelopment of self-identity following emotional trauma (Jochims 1992), encourage a sense of individuality (Bright & Signorelli 1999) or create a new identity (Price-Lackey & Cashman 1996).

Choice of music therapy method

In the literature, there is limited discussion of strategies in choosing appropriate music therapy methods at the beginning of therapy. Given the variety of possible interventions, we have to ask ourselves, 'How do music therapists choose which methods are appropriate for their clients?' We see in Table 2.1 the variety of musical-based interventions possible in neurological rehabilitation.

Baker (2001, p.188) mentions an 'ongoing music therapy debate about the appropriateness of live and taped music in treatment protocols'. Her research demonstrates that patients show a preference for listening to live music and attain better recall of the live presentation of music than recorded music. In response to this she states:

> With respect to music therapy practise, both live and taped music may have their advantages and a place in practice. Taped music is the easier mode to administer and hospital staff could be trained to implement the programs at appropriate times when the music therapist may be unavailable. (ibid.)

Thus the use of recorded music in the treatment of people with post-traumatic amnesia may be a therapeutic strategy that is available to many professionals and not restricted to trained music therapists.

Table 2.1 Music-based interventions used with varying age groups in neurological rehabilitation settings predominantly with TBI

Age group	Reference	Music therapy technique
Children	Tamplin, J. 2000	Improvisation
	Bischof, S. 2001	Improvisation
	Kennelly, J., Hamilton, L. & Cross, J. 2001	Joint treatment with speech pathologist, song singing, song creation, improvised song
	Rosenfeld, J. & Dun, B. 1999	Song listening, song singing alongside instrumental improvisation, physical stimulation
	Kennelly, J. & Edwards, J. 1997	Song singing, song creation, improvised song
Children & *adolescents*	Robb, S. 1996	Improvisational song writing, songs used for discharge from hospital
	Emich, I. 1980	Intonation exercises
Children & *adults*	Gilbertson, S. 1999	Improvisation
Adolescents	Noda, R. *et al.* 2003	Musico-kinetic therapy
	Burke, D. *et al.* 2000	Song writing, song listening, song quizzes, instrument playing
	Wit, V.*et al.*, R. 1994	Electro-acoustic music for training attention
	Glassman, L. 1991	Song reminiscing and song text writing, alongside bibliotherapy
	Hiller, P. 1989	Song story
Adolescents *& adults*	Jochims, S. 1990	Improvisation
	Gervin, A. 1991	Song lyrics during dressing
Adults	Price-Lackey, P. & Cashman, J. 1996	'Playing music' (alongside various other activities)
	Paul, S. & Ramsey, D. 2000	Accompaniment to physical or occupational therapy
	Hohmann, W. 1987	Auditive music therapy
	Schinner, K. *et al.* 1995	Auditory stimulation
	Wheeler, B., Shiflett, S. & Nayak, S. 2003	Group/individual music therapy

Age group	Reference	Music therapy technique
Adults cont.	Gadomski, M. & Jochims, S. 1986	Improvisation
	Claeys, M. *et al.* 1989	Improvisation
	Barker, V. & Brunk, B. 1991	Improvisation
	Herkenrath, A. 2002	Improvisation
	Jochims, S. 1992	Improvisation
	Jochims, S. 1994	Improvisation
	Bright, R. & Signorelli, R. 1999	Improvisation
	Nayak, S. *et al.* 2000	Improvisation
	Robinson, G. 2001	Improvisation
	Gilbertson, S. 2002	Improvisation
	Magee, W. & Davidson, J. 2002	Improvisation singing
	Lee, K. & Baker, F. 1997	Instructional song, song composition, creation of 'song-portfolio'
	Magee, W. 1999	Modified melodic intonation therapy, improvisation mentioned
	Carlisle, B. 2000	Music and relaxation therapy versus verbal relation therapy
	Baker, F. 2001	Music reception
	Jones, R. *et al.* 1994	Music reception, non-musical acoustic stimuli
	Oyama, A. *et al.* 2003	Musico-kinetic therapy
	Yamamoto, K. *et al.* 2003	Musico-kinetic therapy
	Jones, C. 1990	No formal method: music reception
	Hurt, C. *et al.* 1998	Rhythmic auditory stimulation
	Cohen, N. 1992	Singing instruction, vocal exercise, physical exercise, breathing exercise, song singing
	Livingston, F. 1996	Singing, song composition, breathing techniques, melodic exercises, playing instruments
	Baker, F. & Wigram, T. 2004	Song singing, vocal exercises
	Tucek, G. *et al.* 2001	Traditional Oriental Music Therapy
	Lucia, C. 1987	Vocalization, song singing, rhythmic speech exercises
All age groups	Purdie, H. 1997	Active, receptive
	Knox, R. & Jutai, J. 1996	Music reception

Uncertainties about the effectiveness of different music therapy methods have been expressed in the study by Magee and Davidson, who come to the conclusion that 'the type of therapy may not be the critical determinant in mood change' (Magee & Davidson 2002, p.26).

The question still remains, 'How is it possible to determine differences between treatment strategies when we do not yet know the specific effects of each of the treatments?' At this stage of development basic research on existing treatment strategies is needed before we begin to carry out comparative studies.

Multidisciplinary approach to rehabilitation

Some authors suggest that a multidisciplinary approach is necessary in rehabilitation with people who have experienced traumatic brain injury (Kennelly, Hamilton & Cross 2001; Paul & Ramsey 2000; Lee & Baker 1997). All of these authors emphasize that this approach is not simply a multiprofessional provision of a variety of therapies, but a unified strategy that fuses therapy-specific methods in attaining shared rehabilitation issues.

Potential benefits of music therapy

Music therapy first appeared in a publication related to rehabilitation with people who have experienced traumatic brain injury in 1980 (Emich 1980). During the 1990s there was an increase in reports of the application of music therapy in neurosurgical and neurological rehabilitation settings. These studies provide varying levels of evidence and information about the potential positive benefits of music therapy in neurorehabilitation. Specific core aspects of music therapy with people who have experienced TBI are apparent from the literature (Gilbertson 2005). These are:

- Music therapy provides a unique non-verbal assessment strategy in initial phases of rehabilitation following TBI.

- Music therapy offers musical dialogue-based interaction for patients emerging from coma or who are initially diagnosed as 'minimally responsive'.

- Music, in a therapeutic setting, is an integrative medium that provides a logical context for initial attempts towards orientation and cognition following trauma.

- Music therapy provides a strategy to enhance memory of events and information during phases of post-traumatic amnesia and neuropsychological disorder.

- Music therapy leads to improvements in vocal ability and some aspects of speech ability including voice control, intonation, rate of speech and verbal intelligibility.

- In therapy music provides an adequate field of interaction for emotional expression, communication of feelings and validation of emotionality.

- Music therapy offers a strategy to positively influence mood state, often affected by TBI.

- Music therapy can lead to an increase in the level of involvement in therapy and rehabilitation in general.

- By focusing on social and psychological areas, music therapy enhances rehabilitation success and, in turn, provides a balance to therapies focused on physical function.

- Music has been used in therapy to positively influence gait, particularly with patients presenting a static level of disability.

- Music therapy is appropriate for patients of many ages, and has been applied with patients from 3 to 84 years of age.

- Music therapy provides a unique therapeutic possibility with patients with severe TBI (Glasgow Coma Score 3–8).

- Music therapy can lead to an increase in independence in activities of daily life.

- People who have experienced TBI have used music therapy to redevelop some aspects of their personal identity.

- Music therapy may offer a relevant and appropriate therapeutic resource in the future for family members of people with TBI.

These potential benefits provide a basis for specific clinical studies. It remains to be seen if music therapy has the discipline to begin such a series of studies. What will be necessary is a coordinated strategy of research. Though changes are required in the collection and measurement of evidence of change, a variety of areas in which music therapy plays a valuable role towards reaching these rehabilitation goals have been identified.

Whereas many therapy strategies in neurorehabilitation focus on regaining functional ability, the application of music therapy can facilitate improvements in both functional and psychosocial aspects of life of people who have experienced TBI. It is an important component of integrative medicine. As we saw in a study of multiple sclerosis (Aldridge 2005; Schmid & Aldridge 2004), while no functional improvements were evident, there were significant changes in self-esteem and reductions in anxiety and depression. Furthermore, the participants regarded themselves no longer as 'sick' but as active creative people.

What we face in terms of research is finding an adequate form of study design. While it is something of a fad within music therapy currently to emphasize systematic reviews and meta-analysis, we cannot do this here because we have no systematic large-scale studies nor comparative data sets. However, what is more troublesome is that some music therapy researchers are failing to understand the difference between a disease, with a recognized pathogen (like tuberculosis), and a syndrome, which is a collective of identifying clinical signs and symptoms that are indicative of a disorder like TBI. We have to perform the basic clinical research first and that will necessitate a research strategy that embraces the variety of approaches that we have in the profession.

What is holding music therapy back is that, although there has been an impressive breadth of pioneer work in this field, those pioneers have established their own interventions and have not established a united or coherent approach. In trying to establish the validity of music therapy in medical settings, there has been an over-emphasis on functional measures and a neglect of what music therapy can bring in terms of psychological and social benefits.

What is also disturbing in many studies of music therapy is that the music is neglected. This approach is not simply the considered application of ordered frequencies in time to promote the recovery of abilities but an intended mutual performance of music as an aesthetic experience in a therapeutic setting. Of course, as it is a form of therapy we should be submitted to the necessary scrutiny for assessing health care delivery but at the same time we need to understand how people respond to *music* as an art form (Aldridge 1996).

Finally, the precipitous leap from a few studies to systematic reviews has ignored the necessary stages in between that will provide suitable material for review. All this points to a general lack of a research strategy to eventually provide the profession with a corpus of knowledge. Although we have moved from the brave pioneer days of music therapy, and those pioneers have now become well-known names, we have replicated this with the same pattern of a new generation of heroic pioneering researchers making names for themselves. While this may be personally gratifying, what the profession needs is for therapists and researchers to have some sense of a coherent research endeavour where we can combine initiatives in a common direction. To do this we need a step by step approach. We can take our different research approaches, but what we need are common goals and a unifying strategy.

CHAPTER 3

Therapeutic Narrative Analysis: How We Look at Cases

The music therapy approach here is based on 'creative music therapy', after Nordoff and Robbins (1977). In this approach, the client, or patient, and the music therapist take part in music improvisation. This is a form of active music therapy that encourages the active role of all participants. Creative music therapy has been used in individual and group music therapy with children and adults (Aldridge 1996; Ansdell 1995; Bruscia 1991; Lee 1996; Wigram, Nygaard Pedersen & Bonde 2002). This current study focuses on individual music therapy.

In the following short excerpt, David Aldridge (1996, p.58) explains the essence of this form of therapy:

> In creative music therapy lies the possibility of hearing, in a dynamic way, the individual as a whole self as well as in relationship with another person. We can hear the person coming into being as he or she creates a relationship in time. In addition music therapy offers the individual a chance to experience the self in time concretely, to hear his or her own self literally coming into being. If human survival is concerned with a repertoire of flexible coping responses to both external and internal demands, then we may hear in the playing of improvised music the creative way in which a person meets those demands. It could be that illness is a state where there is (a) a restriction in the ability of the person to improvise creatively

(i.e., develop new solutions to problems), or (b) a limited repertoire of coping responses. By promoting creative coping responses we may be establishing the possibilities for renewed health. These are based on the creative qualities of the whole person that promote autonomy.

Therapeutic narrative analysis

The research method adopted in this study is known as therapeutic narrative analysis (Aldridge & Aldridge 2002, 2007) and is a form of case study research (Aldridge 2004a). In this book the case is neurological early rehabilitation of traumatic brain injury. The analysis is based on three stories using 12 episodes from music therapy, but the case itself is music therapy intervention in early neurological rehabilitation.

Case study research

The case study is

> a well established research strategy where the focus is on a case (which is interpreted very widely to include the study of an individual person, a group, a setting, an organization, etc) in its own right, and taking its context into account. (Higgins 1993, p.178)

Case study has also been described as 'a way of investigating an empirical topic by following a set of pre-specified procedures' (Yin 1994, p.15). These pre-specified procedures are 'the logical sequence that connects the empirical data to a study's initial research questions and, ultimately, to its conclusions' (ibid., p.19). As mentioned previously, the study here is based on 12 episodes.

The method of therapeutic narrative analysis

Therapeutic narrative analysis is a form of case study research that incorporates elements of the personal construct theory of George Kelly (1955) to elicit categories for the coding of observational events as we see in qualitative research design (Strauss & Corbin 1998). The method focuses on eliciting the meanings we use to understand the world. Those elicited meanings that we give to events are based upon empirical material and are composed of constructs, which become bundled together as categories.

This initial empirical material is video-recorded episodes taken from clinical practice. The basic form is a structured observational approach. As Aldridge describes:

> this approach does not concern itself with identifying a normative pattern, rather it makes explicit idiosyncratic meanings. However, while each set of meanings is personal, and therefore unique, there is built into the theory awareness that we live in shared cultures and that we can share experiences and meanings with others. (1996, p.126)

As we will see later, the musical improvisations are unique but the form of their interpretation, as a musical score, is one form common to our Western musical cultures.

The method has a flexible design, meaning it may include qualitative and quantitative data. Therapeutic narrative analysis is hermeneutic; it is 'based on understanding the meaning of what happens to us in the process of therapy and how we make sense of the world' (Aldridge & Aldridge 2002, p.2). This method is well suited for such a study as it has been developed to enable enquiry into how a creative arts therapist makes sense of processes of change in therapy. Given the nature of traumatic brain injury, the case study methodology fits the clinical picture in that each injury is unique, as is the process of rehabilitation.

There are five phases involved in therapeutic narrative analysis (see Table 3.1).

Table 3.1 Five phases of therapeutic narrative analysis (adapted from Aldridge & Aldridge 2002)

Phase 1	Identify the narrative
Phase 2	Define the ecology of ideas and settings:
	Context 1: The location of ecology of ideas in the existing literature
	Context 2: The setting in which the narrative occurred
Phase 3	Identify the episodes (select episodes that illustrate the focus of interest) and generate categories
Phase 4	Submit the episodes to analysis
Phase 5	Explicate the research narrative

In Phase 1 we are asked to identify the narrative to be researched. The narrative is the story we wish to investigate. In this study the narrative is about change in music therapy with three individuals who have experienced traumatic brain injury.

Phase 2 is concerned with positioning this narrative in the context of the ecology of ideas in existing literature. This phase is presented in the literature review in Chapter 2.

In Phase 3 episodes are selected that illustrate the focus of interest. This means that the therapist is asked to make choices about the significance of events that have taken place in music therapy. The therapist also makes decisions about which patients will be considered in the study. In his discussion of case study designs, Aldridge (2004a) suggests the term 'reality sampling' to describe the process of selecting patients from clinical experience. In contrast to experimental or controlled studies he emphasizes that 'Many of us have to be content with the people that we meet in practice as the population of our sample' (ibid., p.11). In a process of comparative descriptions, terms are elicited from the therapist to portray similarities or differences between the episodes. These terms reflect the therapist's construing and are referred to as constructs. At a further level of abstraction categories are then elicited from the constructs. Categories have been defined as 'concepts, derived from data, that stand for phenomena' (ibid., p.114).

Constructs lead the researcher to identify core categories at a higher level of abstraction. A core category expresses the main focus of the 'story', relating the constructs and categories to their underlying theory (Strauss & Corbin 1998). Dey describes how

> Selecting a core category seems to involve the elimination of alternative accounts – for these are relegated to future reports. It suggests that there is no place for conflicting and contradictory explanations, which may be more or less supported by the available evidence. (1999, p.112)

The sources of core categories, also referred to as 'central categories' (Strauss & Corbin 1998), are twofold:

A central category may evolve out of the list of existing categories.
Or, a researcher may study the categories and determine that,

although each category tells part of the story, none captures it completely. Therefore, another more abstract term or phrase is needed, a conceptual idea under which all the other categories can be subsumed. (p.146)

Strauss provides criteria for the selection of a core category in that they have a central explanatory power; that within all or almost all cases, there are indicators pointing to that concept; the category is logical and consistent; and the name or phrase used to describe the central category should be sufficiently abstract leading to the development of a more general theory. One should also be able to explain contradictory or alternative cases in terms of the central idea based on the core categories (Strauss 1987).

Phase 4 is concerned with analysing the episodes using a musicological analysis of transcribed representations of the musical events in the episodes. Using these techniques it is possible to describe the episodes in terms of musical change. These analyses are supported by descriptions of the episodes using the elicited constructs and categories. We will see these analyses in Chapters 4, 5 and 6.

In Phase 5 the researcher explicates or clarifies the meaning of the narrative in terms of the results of the analysis. It is this phase that aims at making the construing of the therapist transparent and coherent as understanding. This will be the basis of Chapter 7.

Selecting episodes and archiving video material

At the time of data collection and the archiving of the videotapes there was no systematic process based on clear-cut selection criteria for the deleting and saving of video footage to be used. The videotaped material was collected as a standard part of everyday clinical practice (with patient/caregiver consent). In fact, within the practice of music therapy, we are not aware of the existence of any formalized or standardized criteria for the deletion and saving of video footage in clinical practice, although a considerable debate is taking place in qualitative research in international nursing circles.

Although formalized criteria do not exist, practical and pragmatic reasons have determined why some recordings of therapy are saved and others are deleted. Video and audio recordings of therapy sessions, or selections of these sessions, have been retained that are of clinical interest in the therapeutic process or demonstrate aspects of 'standard clinical practice' at the time of recording. Some of these recordings are saved specifically for demonstration purposes within the multidisciplinary team, some in the form of anecdotal case studies, or to provide feedback to patients and their families. At the time of archiving, it was usual practice in the clinic to delete all recordings of therapy that were not retained based on the aforementioned reasons. As this is a retrospective study, we could only use what was to hand. However, in terms of qualitative research a selection had already taken place, as those examples were retained that were relevant as examples significant for clinical practice.

After repeated viewing of the remaining video recordings, 63 excerpts were chosen for closer viewing. These excerpts were selected as they demonstrated significant events of therapeutic change as judged by the therapist. This form of sampling is referred to as purposive (Robson 2002, p.193) and is undertaken to generate conceptual categories. Robson and qualitative researchers often mention this generation of categories as if it is a natural occurrence. But for any everyday qualitative researcher, there are few examples of how exactly to generate these categories, rather than relying upon pulling them from out of the air. Therapeutic narrative analysis incorporates personal construct methodology to elicit those tacit understandings we have as constructs. These constructs can then be bundled together as categories, thus offering the reader a backward chain of evidence showing how those categories, were achieved.

To reduce the number of episodes originating from the same case, each of the rough episodes were compared in their level of similarity. Where similarities in the observed events exist, the choice to retain or discard an excerpt was made based on the following two questions:

1. Does the episode clearly demonstrate the type of event targeted?

2. Does the episode illustrate an event more clearly in the therapy process when compared to a similar excerpt?

Based on these steps, 12 episodes were selected from the 63 rough episodes for analysis.

These coarse episodes were then reduced to specific episodes as an initial form of categorization in qualitative research. An episode is a finer time selection, a reduction that precisely covers the targeted material, in this case the behavioural or musical activity. Categorization in qualitative research is based on a conceptual abstraction. In a music therapy research sense, this categorization from coarse episode to episode, for future repertory grid analysis, is made from aural and visual modalities and not simply textual. The 12 episodes are taken from individual music therapy with three individuals, Bert, Neil and Mark (names changed). Each episode is given a unique name, hinting at what happened in the event recorded (see Table 3.2).

Table 3.2 The 12 episodes and their episode names, participants and duration

Episode number	Episode name	Participant	Duration (minutes.seconds)
Episode 1	First foot forward	Bert	00.53
Episode 2	Long Indian phrase		02.20
Episode 3	Touching foot		02.02
Episode 4	Foot cymbal		01.28
Episode 5	Crying	Neil	01.17
Episode 6	Hello Neil		00.38
Episode 7	From behind the covers		01.32
Episode 8	Hello Simon		01.34
Episode 9	Light in a dark night	Mark	02.48
Episode 10	The flute is my voice		01.50
Episode 11	Steel drum		02.20
Episode 12	9th September		02.27

Constructing categories

Once the episodes have been selected constructs are elicited by considering three of the episodes and describing why two of the episodes are similar and how the remaining episode is different (see Aldridge 1996).

The constructs are bipolar and may be single words or short phrases. The therapist is required to rank the remaining episodes somewhere along a continuum between the constructs in a manner that makes sense to him/her (Figure 3.1). The rankings of the episodes represent the relationship between the episodes in terms of the constructs. This elicitation provides a means for the therapist to express thoughts in a form accessible for others. As Aldridge and Aldridge (2002, p.10) state: 'The verbalization of musical experiences is one step on the way to establishing credibility by getting the practitioner to say what he or she means in his or her own words.'

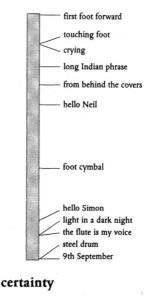

Figure 3.1 Ranking episodes along the continuum of constructs

The process of eliciting constructs using RepGrid is carried out in a conversational interaction between researcher and mentor. This means the researcher and the supervisor talk together about the researcher's construing. By doing this step together the eliciting of constructs has taken place in discourse and 'this negotiating of a common sense is a part of the supervisory activity and the ground for establishing validity in a qualitative paradigm' (Aldridge & Aldridge 2002, p.11).

The constructs elicited through the comparison of the episodes are shown in Table 3.3.

Table 3.3 Constructs elicited from comparison of the episodes

harmonic simplicity	harmonic complexity
simple timbre	complex timbre
small utterance	extended play
making sounds	making music
questionable	certainty
isolated actions	integrated actions
being directive	non-directive
responding	initiating
being led	leading
distress	calm
vocal	instrumental
conventional use of instrument	individual use of instrument
occurs in and out	specific to music therapy (MT)

The process of eliciting constructs and the ranking of episodes has been carried out using the RepGrid software (RepGrid 2 V.2.1b, Centre for Person-Computer Studies, Calgary, Canada). The RepGrid software was designed to document the process of eliciting constructs and the ranking of the episodes in terms of the constructs by the researcher. The RepGrid software produces two forms of data analysis and representation. To create a spatial representation of the constructs and episodes, the values given to the episodes are organized by similarities and represented in clusters on two principal axes. This graphic representation is known as principal components analysis. The axes themselves are generated from the data and as yet have no name. As we will see later, in Chapter 7, these two principal axes will become important for understanding the rest of the data.

The principal components analysis is shown below in Figure 3.2. This representation shows correlations between episodes and the construct pairs through the position of the episode and constructs. The episodes are marked with an x beside the episode name.

RepGrid also provides a representation of the constructs in matrix form (Figure 3.3). This computation is known as focus analysis. In this mode, we see how the therapist has rank ordered the episodes. The focus analysis provides an additional perspective where 'clusters of constructs are then computed by selecting the most similar ratings and presented as a hierarchical tree diagram that shows linkages between groups of constructs' (Aldridge & Aldridge 2002, p.12). The groupings of constructs are then given labels that 'themselves represent constructs at a greater level of abstraction. The labels are a step in finding categories for use in analysing case material in qualitative research' (ibid.).

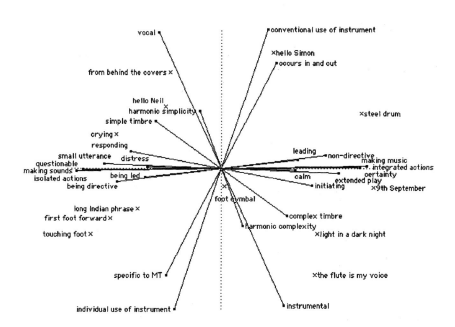

Figure 3.2 Principal components analysis created with RepGrid

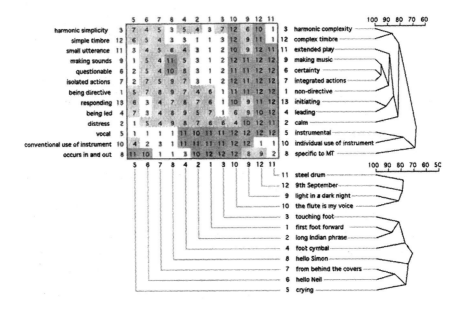

Figure 3.3 Focus analysis of the 12 episodes in RepGrid

The categories

Note: In all the following sections, the *constructs* are marked in italics and **categories** are marked in bold.

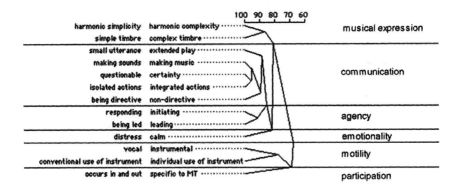

Figure 3.4 The constructs and categories elicited using RepGrid

The focus analysis shows the correlations between constructs as a tree-diagram to the right of the constructs (see Figure 3.4 marked as a scale 100–60). The correlations suggest groupings of constructs. From these groupings, the following categories have been elicited: **musical expression, communication, agency, emotionality, motility** and **participation** (see Figure 3.4).

Musical expression

The category **musical expression** is derived from the two construct pairs *harmonic simplicity/harmonic complexity* and *simple timbre/complex timbre*.

In his discussion of the term 'expression' Scruton (1999, p.155) states:

> Granted that we spontaneously extend our mental predicates to music, what need have we of the term 'express'? Is there any difference between the judgement that a work is sad, and the judgement that it expresses sadness? *Both* of these descriptions are metaphorical: hence we can use them to make the same point, or different points, depending on the context. Nevertheless, the use of the term 'express' seems to imply human agency of some kind, and also the attempt to articulate something.

If musical expression is an indicator of an 'attempt to articulate something' we may consider the musical parameters that are used to demonstrate musical expression as indicators of how music is heard. These musical parameters are metaphors for the interpretation of how the music has been heard:

> Expression and expressiveness here coincide – an interesting fact that tells us something about our interest in expression. The expressive word or gesture is the one that awakens our sympathy, the one that invites us into a mental orbit that is not our own. If we think that all artistic expression is also expressive, that is surely a fact about how we respond to expression in art. It is plausible to suppose, therefore, that a theory of expression must incorporate a theory of our response to it. (Scruton 1999, p.154)

The term 'musical expression' is used here to describe what is heard and how the listener has given meaning to it.

Communication

The category **communication** has been derived from the construct pairs *small utterance/extended play, making sounds/making music, questionable/certainty, isolated actions/integrated action* and *being directive/non-directive.*

'Communication' derives from the Latin verb *communicare*, 'to share'. The verb 'communicate' has been defined as 'to share or exchange information, news, or ideas'. A further usage of the term 'communicate' is to 'convey or transmit (an emotion or a feeling) in a non-verbal way' (Soanes & Stevenson 2003). This usage highlights the possibility of transferring meaning without using words. Scruton (1999, p.18) suggests:

> Every sound intentionally made is instinctively taken to be an attempt at communication. And this is as true of music as it is of speech. In the presence of sound intentionally produced, and intentionally organized, we feel ourselves within another person's ambit. And that feeling conditions our response to what we hear.

The term 'communication' includes both the transfer and sharing of information and meaning, and the transmission of emotions and feelings.

Agency

The category **agency** has been derived from the construct pairs *responding/initiating* and *being led/leading.*

'Agency' has been defined as 'the operation or action of an agent' where an 'agent' is defined 'as a person or thing that exerts power' (Kirkpatrick 1983). Its Latin root *agere* means 'doing'. This is a central point in creative music therapy, as it is not simply one person doing music to another but two people doing music together as performance. For the people here, after an accident, the idea that they can do something, to achieve personal agency, no matter how brief or small, is a central plank in their recovery to autonomy.

The term 'agency' is used to relate to situations in which a person is able to exert power or influence that leads to a particular result.

Emotionality

The category **emotionality** has been derived from the construct pair *distress/calm*. The term 'emotionality' stems from the term 'emotional', which has been defined as 'arousing or characterized by intense feeling' (Soanes & Stevenson 2003). If something is described as emotional then it relates to our emotions. Emotion is defined as 'a strong feeling deriving from one's circumstances, mood, or relationships with others' (Soanes & Stevenson 2003). The term is rooted in the Latin word *movere*, meaning 'move'. This sense of moving is commonly used in modern language, as in the phrase 'the piece of music was very moving'. This may refer to 'moving' between various emotional states. However, as we will see in the next category, moving and motility are interlinked. Indeed, it may be that what is moving in music is a powerful motivator to achieve motility, providing the necessary energy to achieve it. Remember that the people we are talking about here have been in severe accidents that have left them very disabled.

Motility

The category **motility** has been derived from the construct pairs *vocal /instrumental* and *conventional use of instrument/individual use of instrument*.

The term 'motility' derives from the Latin word *motus*, meaning 'motion'. Motion is defined as 'the action or process of being moved' (Soanes & Stevenson 2003). The term 'motion' is also defined in the sense of a gesture (Soanes & Stevenson 2003), such as 'to make a motion with the hand'. Motility is used to refer to the ability to make a motion or gesture.

In practice, what we are often asked by family and friends is 'Will he ever move again?' and then, 'Will she ever speak again?' A precursor to movement and to the achievement of language is gesture. In our earlier study of child development it was hand–eye coordination that became central and necessary for the achievement of cognitive abilities. Being able to gesture and convert that gestural impulse into a movement that beats an instrument within a context of musical time is critical for the achievement of both physical and mental coherence for the person them-selves and for their communication with others.

Participation

The category **participation** derives from the construct pair *occurs in and out/specific to music therapy.*

The etymological background of the term 'participation' lies in the Latin term *participare*, based on *pars*, meaning 'part', and *capere*, meaning 'take'. The modern definition of the term 'participation' is 'the action of taking part in something' (Soanes & Stevenson 2003). Participation is a central theme in creative music therapy. It is also the necessary precursor for rehabilitation. All therapists will need the active participation of the patient. Even in research we now write of participants, not of subjects, emphasizing the active agency of the person.

Coda

Anyone working in this field will know that there are very profound questions being asked by family and friends. 'Will he walk again?', 'Will she ever smile?', 'Does she know we are here?' All these embrace the categories presented here of **communication**, **agency**, **motility** and **participation**. Combined with these categories of autonomy and relationship we also have expressive qualities of **musical expression** and **emotionality**. Being able to express ourselves in a relationship, to communicate our needs and establish a mutuality of meaning, is central for establishing our autonomy and for maintaining meaningful relationships. This promotion of meaningful expression is an important part of rehabilitation. It is not simply functional but reflects what it is to be a functional human being.

In the next three chapters we will see how these categories emerge based on musical examples and what the ramifications are for the process of rehabilitation.

CHAPTER 4

Bert's Story: Changing Perspectives – Identifying and Realizing Communicative Potential in Early Isolated States

A car collided with Bert as he was riding his bicycle. Bert was 14 years old at the time. As a result of this incident he sustained severe traumatic brain injury with multiple contusions, bleeding and haemorrhages. His skull was fractured as well as both his legs. Following emergency surgical treatment he was transferred to intensive care. Later, he required reconstructive neurosurgery to the skull and the implantation of an artificial feeding tube through his nose as he was unable to swallow.

Nine weeks after the traumatic event Bert was admitted to Klinik Holthausen. At this time he presented unstable vegetative functions, an extreme increase of muscle tone in all extremities, inconsistent spontaneous head and leg movement, and responded to pain with undirected minimal movement. He did not speak, and he was described as presenting characteristics of apallic syndrome.[1]

Bert opened his eyes without focusing on any person or object, and his eyes showed divergent and convergent movement. He did not follow

---

[1]   Apallic syndrome is a term often used in Europe similar to persistent vegetative state and its use is still in debate.

any movement with his eyes but did show a questionable pupil reaction to light in his left eye. At this time Bert reacted to being spoken to with increased tonus of the extremities. He did move his mouth, but this was considered to be a reflex. His physical movement was restricted to occasional spontaneous head movement, discrete movement of his hands and feet, and a massive increase in muscle tone of all extremities and the neck.

Bert began individual music therapy at the beginning of August, 16 weeks post-trauma. He initially received physiotherapy, balneotherapy,[2] intensive nursing and music therapy followed by speech therapy. For the duration of his treatment he received a wide range of medication to relieve his spasms and prevent any seizures.

Episode 1: 'First foot forward'

Episode 1 is selected from the second music therapy session with Bert. The therapist plays piano and the patient has a single row of wind chimes positioned above his left foot. The wind chimes are so placed that if Bert should raise his foot, the chimes move and make their characteristic sound. At the time of the recording, many therapists and nurses had observed Bert's foot rising and falling, bending at his knee joint. After a few days of observation, it was suggested that this movement had no meaning and was an uncoordinated impulse.[3] In any case, the therapists involved did not see this activity as having any therapeutic potential. Bert was receiving physiotherapy, occupational therapy, speech therapy (in the form of oral stimulation, not speech rehabilitation), nursing care and medication.

Though there was a high level of uncertainty about Bert's movements, something very significant happened in this first episode. We started to ask, 'What links the patient's actions and the music played by the therapist?' Though it was not possible to answer immediately, the posing of the question was central. It was necessary to 'do' the question and not to attempt to answer it theoretically. Aldridge's perspective on science is that of doing knowledge. We test out our hypotheses in

2   Balneotherapy is a form of spa treatment involving baths and various herbal and mineral preparations.

3   For a further discussion of such movements being dismissed as having no meaning see A. Herkenrath in Aldridge 2005.

practice. If Bert moves, and this can be made sense of within the musical playing, then we demonstrate intention.

The transcription of the events shows Bert's foot movement, the sounding of the wind chimes, and the music played by the therapist on the piano. A harmonic analysis is presented on the lower stave, called 'Middle ground'.

The signs used in the music transcription of Episode 1 are shown in Figure 4.1.

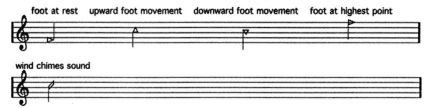

Figure 4.1 Signs used in the transcription of Episode 1

In the principal components analysis (see Figure 3.2), Episode 1 appears near to the constructs *being led,* from the category **agency**, *being directive, isolated actions, making sounds* and *questionable,* from the category **communication**, and *specific to music therapy,* from the category **participation**.

In this episode (Figure 4.2) the therapist is *being directive* and leads the improvisation on the piano; the patient remains still and does not move. It is only at the close of the episode that the patient moves his foot into the wind chimes in a single *isolated action.* The therapist is unsure whether the patient is making music; it is suggested that he may only be *making sounds,* not being directly aware of the musical implications of his playing. Though the actions of the therapist and patient seem coordinated, the episode is characterized by an uncertainty and the patient's awareness of the interaction seems *questionable.* These constructs belong to the category **communication**; the therapist is focused on interaction and communication. The patient is *being led* by the therapist and in this sense the patient's level of **agency** may be limited and it seems that the therapist is determining the course of events.

Episode 1: First foot forward

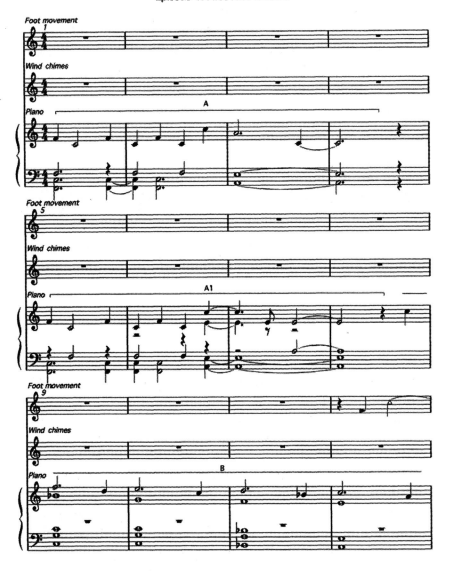

Figure 4.2 Transcription of Episode 1

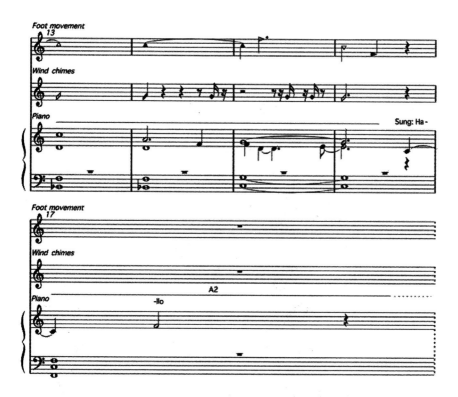

Figure 4.2 Transcription of Episode 1 (continued)

Sonogram

Note: A sonogram shows the intensity of frequencies on the y-axis and over time along the x-axis. The time-code of a sonogram allows the exact description of the relationship of events to each other in time.

Four clear melodic structures can be seen in the sonogram of Episode 1 (Figure 4.3). The tones of the piano melody are marked in the figure with small circles and joined by lines to show the melodic movement. Here we can see similarities between the contours of the first two phrases. Also apparent is the long falling sequence in the third and fourth phrases. The two occasions where the wind chime is sounded is marked with positions Y and X. The wind chimes can be identified by the simultaneous sounding of a wide range of frequencies shown in the sonogram at the time-codes 0:00.37 and 0:00.49.

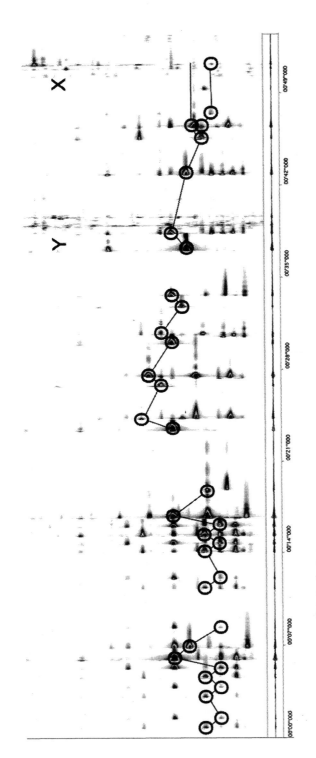

Figure 4.3 Sonogram of Episode 1

Y and X indicate the sounding of the wind chimes; circles mark the piano tones linked by lines to indicate the melody line.

A sonogram is a sound spectrogram or audio spectrogram that displays the energy in a sound plotting the frequency (pitch) of the sound on the vertical axis against time on the horizontal axis. The loudest (amplitude) is represented by the density of the image.

Musicological analysis

This 50-second episode is made up of two short phrases and two longer phrases.

MELODY

The initial melody structure (marked as 'A' in the notation) is characterized by a triadic, four bar phrase. The melody has a range of one octave. There is a clear sense of tonality (F major) that is emphasized by the accompanying chords played in root position. The first phrase (A) is repeated once with some slight variation (A1). The closure of the phrase is changed and, through an earlier sounding of the second chord (A minor) on the fourth beat of the second bar, a sense of immediacy can be felt. By ending on the fifth tone of the dominant minor chord, which is also the leading tone of the tonic chord (F major), the melody tone 'e' creates a pressure of movement upwards and towards resolution on the tone 'f'.

This resolution is implied at the beginning of the third phrase. The third phrase consists of a falling sequence, of eight bars' duration (bars 9 to 16), that leads stepwise down the scale of F major. The melodic completion of this phrase occurs with the cadential resolution at the beginning of the next phrase (bar 17). A suspended dominant chord (bar 15) increases a sense of coming to rest and is resolved on the upbeat to bar 16.

Combining the sonogram and the musical analysis

By comparing the sonogram, melody and video, we see that the patient begins to move his foot at the end of the third phrase played by the therapist, shortly before the therapist plays a suspended cadential chord passage in bar 13. The suspended dominant chord in bar 15 is synchronized with the initial downward movement of the patient's foot and the resolution shortly pre-empts the return of the patient's foot to the position of rest. There is a synchronization of harmonic changes on the piano with the timing of the patient's foot movement. It is *questionable* whether this chord sequence is actually *leading* the patient's actions. It is possible that the therapist is *being led* by the patient's foot movement. As a conclusion, it is unclear who is *being directive* and who is *being led*, and this remains *questionable*. Both players may be showing characteristics of both constructs.

The therapist synchronized the timing of the cadential passage (B) to the patient's movements. This was done to create a meaningful context for the patient's foot movement. The therapist used a suspended dominant chord to freeze the harmonic movement in the music and use a flexible time-stretching function. Consequently the therapist is able to synchronize the resolution of suspended chord with the moment the patient's foot returned to the rest position. This makes sense in music. This synchronization of movement to music is *specific to music therapy*. For the therapist, it was *questionable* whether Bert was aware of the significance of his actions.

Episode 2: 'Long Indian phrase'

Episode 2 is taken from the second music therapy session with Bert. He is sitting with the wind chimes in front of his left foot; the therapist is at the piano.

The episode is characterized by an ostinato figure in the bass of the piano. The tones that are repeatedly played are 'a2', 'e2', 'a3', 'e3' and 'a4' (440 Hz). These tones are played in a rhythmic but not metrical manner and have a drone quality. The music in this episode is not continuously metrically organized, but is rhythmically flexible.

The signs used in the music transcription of Episode 2 are shown in Figure 4.4.

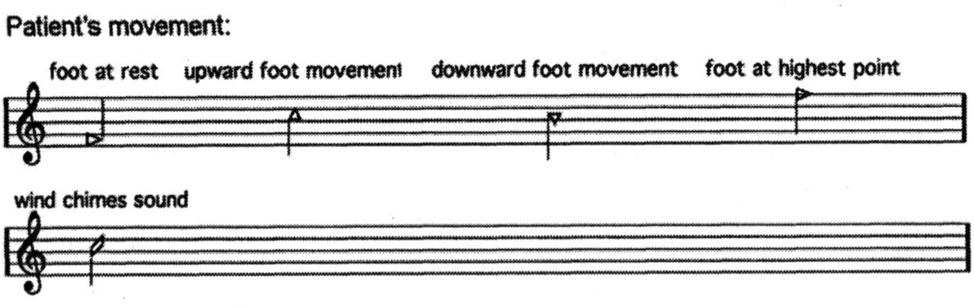

Figure 4.4 Signs used in the transcription of Episode 2

Episode 2 (Figure 4.5) appears near to the constructs *being led, being directive* and *specific to music therapy* in the principal components analysis. These constructs belong to the category **communication**.

Harmonic structure and form

In this episode the therapist plays an ostinato accompaniment figure in the mid-lower range of the piano. This pattern consists of the pitches 'a2', 'e2', 'a3', 'e3' and 'a4'. The ostinato is not metric, but is organized rhythmically.

Melody

After transcribing the pitches of the melodies, the structures of the melodies became transparent (Table 4.1). There is a predominance of falling contours (melodic forms A and C) in the melodic form of the nine melodies. The melodic forms B and D include stepwise upward movement and an interval leap in form B. The melodies are built upon the scale made up of the tones 'a', 'b', 'c', 'd', 'e', 'f' and 'g'. This scale is also known as the hypodorian scale.

Table 4.1 Melodic form of the nine melodies sung by the therapist in Episode 2

Melody	Description	Melodic form
1	Four tone melody moving stepwise from 'a4', 'g4', 'f4', to 'e4'	A
2	Four tone melody moving stepwise from 'a4', 'g4', 'f4', to 'e4'	A
3	Four tone melody initially moving stepwise from 'd4', 'c3', 'b3' and jumping upwards to 'e4'	B
4	Four tone melody moving stepwise from 'a4', 'g4', 'f4', to 'e4'	A
5	Four tone melody moving stepwise from 'd4', 'c3', 'b3', to 'a4'	C
6	Four tone melody moving stepwise from 'g3', 'a3', 'b3', to 'a3'	D
7	Four tone melody moving stepwise from 'g3', 'a3', 'b3', to 'a3'	D
8	Four tone melody moving stepwise from 'a4', 'g4', 'f4', to 'e4'	A
9	Four tone melody moving stepwise from 'a4', 'g4', 'f4' (repeated), to 'e4'	A

Episode 2: Long Indian phrase

Figure 4.5 Transcription of Episode 2

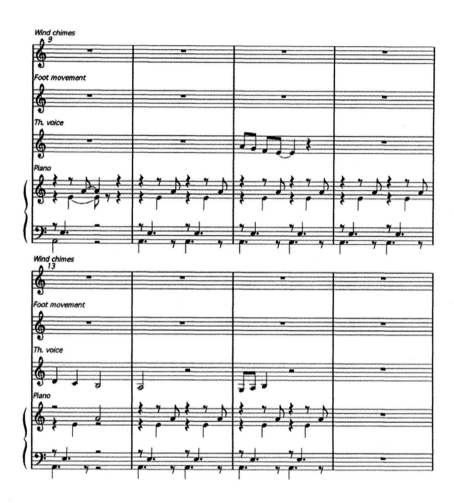

Figure 4.5 Transcription of Episode 2 (continued)

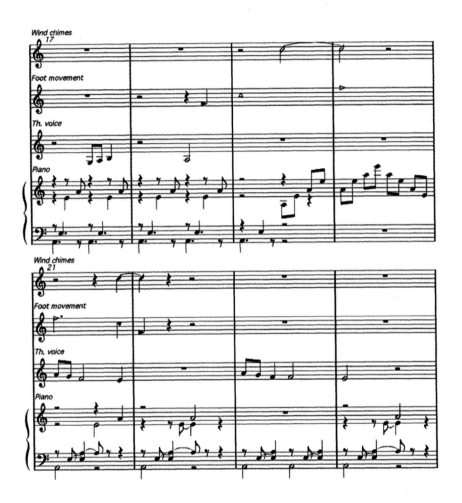

Figure 4.5 Transcription of Episode 2 (continued)

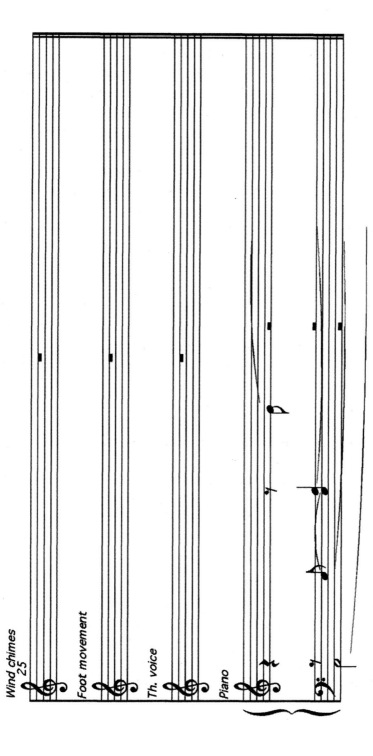

Figure 4.5 Transcription of Episode 2 (continued)

Video analysis

In the video recording of Episode 2 we see a synchronization of the patient's movement and the music played and sung by the therapist. These movements include foot movements, mouth movements and yawning. The therapist's improvising is *being led* by the patient's mouth movements. The therapist synchronizes his singing to these movements and each melody tone begins as the patient opens his mouth (0:00.15–0:00.26). As the patient raises his foot into the wind chimes, the therapist begins singing the first melody (melody 1). After the repetition of this melody (melody 2) comes to a close, the patient lowers his foot to the rest position. The therapist's melodies (melodies 3, 4, 5, 6 and 7) are synchronized to the patient's mouth movements (0:00.27–0:01.25).

In this episode actions are synchronized by 'stretching' time without losing the sense of the structure of the melodic phrases played by the therapist. This form of temporal flexibility may be *specific to music therapy*.

The patient plays the wind chimes for the second time at the end of melody 7. The therapist replies by repeating the initial melody (melody 1) and repeats this melody once again after the patient moves his foot to the rest position. The therapist extends the duration of the penultimate tone of melody 8 to accompany the patient's foot as it returns to the rest position using the repetition of melodic motives to demonstrate a meaningful structure to the patient.

The patient's mouth movements and foot movements may be *isolated* from a normal perspective of communicative interaction yet set in a musical context they become meaningful. The organization of related actions within a meaningful structure is necessary for **communication**.

Episode 3: 'Touching foot'

Episode 3 is taken from the fourth music therapy session with Bert. The therapist plays the piano and Bert has the wind chimes above his left foot.

The transcription shows the music played by the therapist on the piano, the tactile impulses given by the therapist, the movement of the patient's foot and the sounding of the wind chimes. The wind chimes do not directly sound when contacted by the patient's foot movement. It is the synchronization between the patient's movement and the therapist's actions that is of interest in this episode.

The main focus points in this episode are the wind chime playing of the patient with his own foot, the music played on the piano and the touches that the therapist makes to Bert's foot. At one stage (0:00.06), the therapist verbally encourages the patient with an assuring 'yes'. The question of a possible link between these elements lies at the heart of the episode.

The signs used in the music transcription of Episode 3 are shown in Figure 4.6.

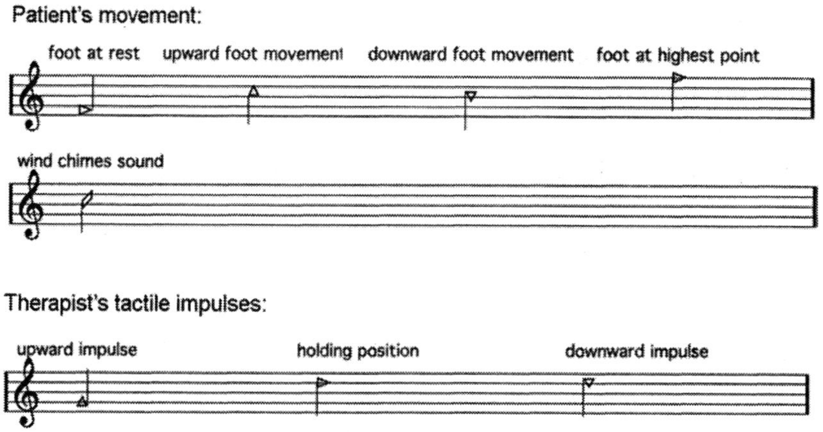

Patient's movement:

Therapist's tactile impulses:

Figure 4.6 Signs used in the transcription of Episode 3

Episode 3 (Figure 4.7) appears in the principal components analysis near to the constructs *being directive, being led* and *isolated actions,* belonging to the category **communication**, *individual use of instrument,* belonging to the category **agency**, and *specific to music therapy,* belonging to the category **participation**.

In the overview of Episode 3 in Figure 4.8 we can see six similar patterns or phrases in the music played by the therapist on the piano (marked with grey squares).

The sounding of the wind chimes, the patient's foot movement and the therapist's tactile impulses take place during the pauses between these phrases. This form suggests organization or the attempt towards organization. At this point the therapist is *being directive.* A particular meaning is

Episode 3: Touching foot

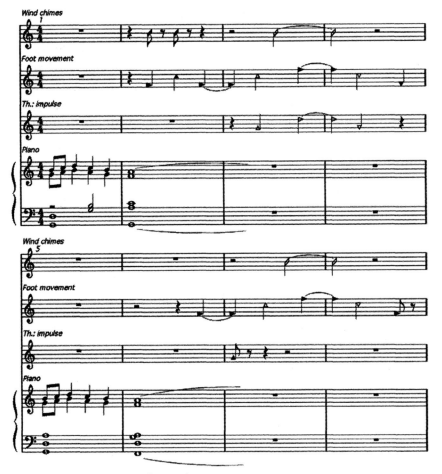

Figure 4.7 Transcription of Episode 3

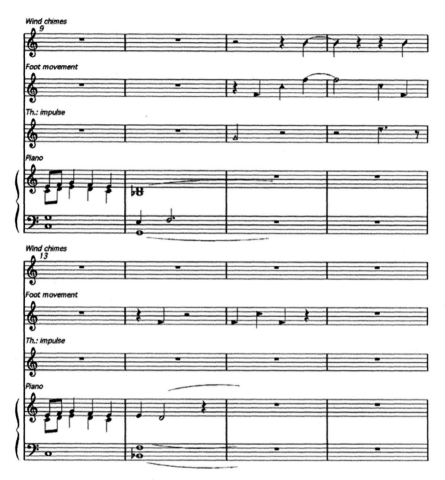

Figure 4.7 Transcription of Episode 3 (continued)

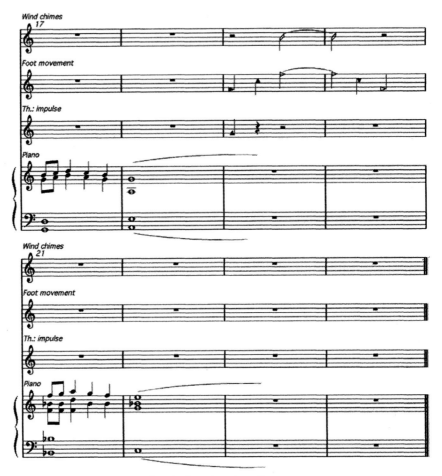

Figure 4.7 Transcription of Episode 3 (continued)

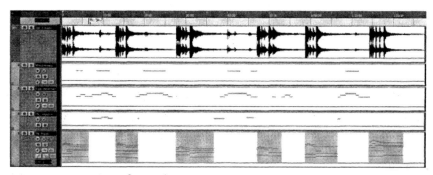

Figure 4.8 Overview of Episode 3

given to the actions of the patient. In this situation the therapist is not only determining what the patient should do, but also suggesting the sense of what is being done in the context. The patient is *being led* within a logical music structure. This logic pertains to cognition, and relies on recognizing the pattern of logic used in the exchange.

There are two events of special interest in this episode. Almost immediately after the final melody tone of the first phrase is played (bars 1 and 2), the patient begins to raise his foot towards the wind chimes. The patient does not reach the wind chimes and his foot returns shortly to rest. The two single wind chime beats heard at the beginning of the episode are caused by earlier actions not seen in the episode. The therapist quickly takes gentle hold of the patient's foot and moves carefully upwards into the wind chimes. After the wind chimes sound he slowly returns the patient's foot to the rest position. This interaction includes two elements: phrases played by the therapist on the piano and the patient moving his foot to play the wind chimes.

After the second phrase played on the piano (bars 5 and 6), the therapist lightly touches the bottom of the patient's foot. The patient moves his leg upwards and makes the wind chimes sound. This pattern repeats once again in bars 9–12. The therapist touches the patient's foot lightly at the beginning of bar 11, suggesting an upwards movement, and in bar 12 to suggest the patient move his foot downwards. The therapist is *leading* the patient in the alternating actions. The patient is *being led* within the alternation of actions.

In the overview in Figure 4.9 we can see a variation in the amount of time passing between each of the phrases played by the therapist (shown with grey squares).

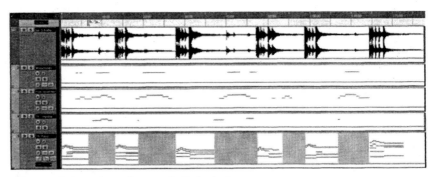

Figure 4.9 Overview of pauses in Episode 3

The pauses following the second, third and fifth piano phrases are clearly longer than the pauses following the other phrases. This suggests some form of waiting, providing Bert with the opportunity to play autonomously. It is reasonable to assume that the therapist is using a model of turn taking that is occurring within boundaries of a flexible temporal organization. The term 'boundary' refers here to the point of time at which the meaning of context may become lost if it is exceeded. These are boundaries of temporal coherence. Shortly before this boundary is reached the therapist becomes active and gives a tactile impulse to the patient's foot.

After the fourth repetition of the piano melody (bars 13 and 14) the patient begins to move his foot upward but, as in bar 2, returns to rest without reaching the wind chimes. On this occasion, in contrast to the first instance, the therapist does not direct the patient to play through tactile impulse. The patient is not *being led* extensively, but has the opportunity for **agency** and may determine that the wind chimes are not played at this point.

The fifth repetition of the melody (bars 17 and 18) is very similar to the second. After a pause the therapist gives a minimal impulse to the underside of the patient's foot. The patient subsequently moves his foot upwards and plays the wind chimes.

The sixth repetition of the melody (bars 21 and 22) mirrors the rhythmic structure of the previous repetitions. It is in a higher register, beginning on the tone 'f4', and follows the same melodic contour as the previous repetitions. After the melody is completed the patient does not play the wind chimes within the same time range as the previous phrases.

The principal components analysis shows proximity between Episode 3 and the construct *specific to music therapy*. This construct has been used to elicit the category **participation**. The patient is showing a *questionable* understanding of his part in the interactions. To participate, others involve us and we take on a part within a social context. In this episode it is possible for the patient to participate in the music therapy activities; at this time these activities are specific to the music therapy context and do not occur outside of this context.

Episode 4: 'Foot cymbal'

Episode 4 is selected from the therapy session on 25 August 1994. The patient is sitting in front of a cymbal. The therapist has placed a drumstick in the patient's elastic trouser-leg. This was necessary for the patient to be able to play the cymbal. The level of spasticity in Bert's arms and hands prohibited him using a drumstick in the conventional manner. In this episode, the therapist sings and plays the piano.

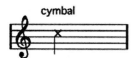

Figure 4.10 Sign used in the transcription of Episode 4

The sign used in the transcription of Episode 4 is shown in Figure 4.10. The principal components analysis shows Episode 4 in the centre of the constellation of all constructs. The episode appears within the bottom right quadrant, and is close to the constructs *calm* and *initiating*, which belong to the categories **emotionality** and **agency**.

In this episode (Figure 4.11), the patient plays on a cymbal hung upside-down, with a drumstick that is resting between his toes and is

Episode 4: Foot cymbal

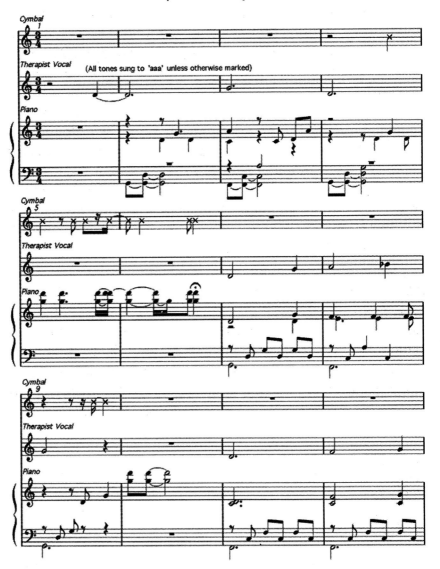

Figure 4.11 Transcription of Episode 4

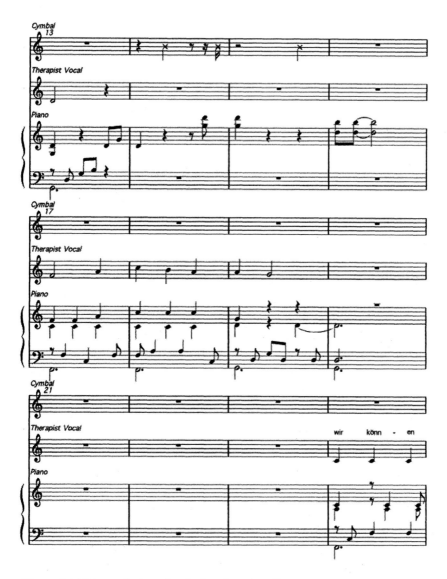

Figure 4.11 Transcription of Episode 4 (continued)

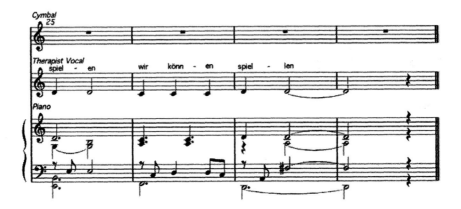

Figure 4.11 Transcription of Episode 4 (continued)

held in place by his elastic trouser-leg. This is an *individual use of instrument*, and describes the state of the patient's **motility**. The principal components analysis shows the episode near *initiating* (from the construct pair *responding/initiating*) and *leading* (from the construct pair *being led/leading*). Both of these constructs are used to define the category **agency**. As we will see, it is possible to identify elements of agency in the musicological analysis.

In the overview (Figure 4.12), we can recognize patterns of alternation between the therapist's singing (bottom) and the patient's cymbal playing (second from top).

The therapist improvises on the piano simultaneously with the patient's cymbal playing (bars 5–6, 9, and 13–14).

There are five distinct phrases in the episode: bars 1–6, 7–10, 11–16, 17–23, and 24–28. The therapist improvises on two harmonies in bars 1–23, G major and F major. In bars 24–28, the therapist uses the chords of F major, E minor and D major. The first four phrases are similar in terms of symmetrical structure of harmony, phrase length and melodic contour.

The barcarolle style of the piano accompaniment, and the small range of harmonic vocabulary, may be responsible for the feeling of **emotionality** that tends towards *calm*. Additionally, the episode is at a quiet

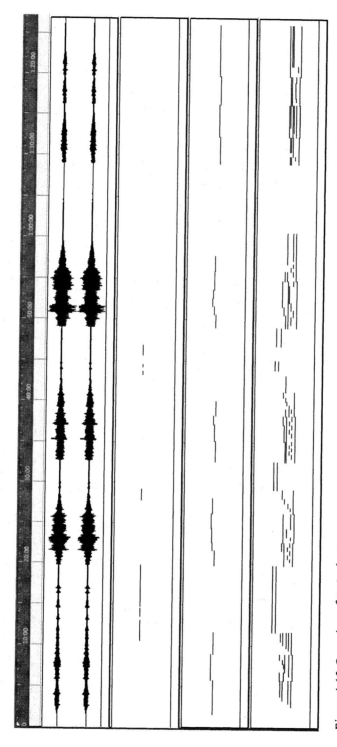

Figure 4.12 Overview of Episode 4

dynamic, between 'mezzo piano' and 'mezzo forte', and the long, held tones sung by the therapist add to the calm atmosphere.

If we look closer at the transcription of Episode 4 we see how the patient is *initiating* rhythmic patterns. This is an important basis for **agency**. The patient and therapist tentatively begin to play simultaneously and show a tendency towards *integrated actions*.

The patient's first cymbal beat occurs on the fourth beat of bar 4. As a consequence, the therapist abruptly ends the pattern he played in the previous three bars and plays a two-tone chord ('g' and 'd') on the first beat of bar 5. The patient's second beat was almost simultaneous with the therapist's first beat of bar 5. The therapist repeats the chord on beat 2 of bar 5, reflecting the two-beat pattern played by the patient, highlighted in the Figure 4.13 with grey squares. On the fourth and fifth quavers of bar 5 the patient reiterates the two-beat pattern, followed by the therapist's answering pattern. The patient begins a new repetition of the two-beat pattern on the last semiquaver of bar 5 and the second quaver beat of bar 6. The therapist does not directly answer this repetition, but waits. The patient and therapist play the two-beat pattern simultaneously on the fourth and fifth quaver beats of bar 6.

Episode 4: Foot cymbal

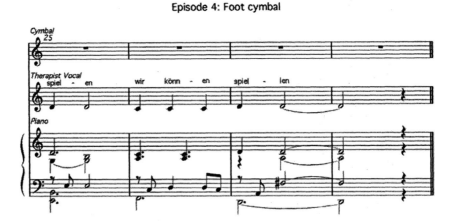

Figure 4.13 Bars 4–6 of Episode 4

In this transcription, we can see the two players in the act of improvising towards a shared understanding, in this excerpt the understanding of a two-note cell. Not only is the content of this cell exchanged, but also synchronization between the players takes place. The improvised music is co-ordinated. Both players are creating order in their co-improvisation.

After the variation (bars 7–9) of the therapist's original phrase, the patient plays a single cymbal beat on the eighth semiquaver beat of bar 9. The therapist plays a two-beat pattern on the first and second quaver beat of bar 10. This two-beat pattern is a citation of the two-beat patterns exchanged in bars 4–7.

The third motive variation (bars 11–13) is followed by a single beat on the cymbal played by the patient. Following a longer pause than in the previous instances, the therapist plays a two-beat pattern on the last quaver of bar 14 and the first quaver of bar 15. In the middle of this pattern the patient plays a single cymbal beat followed by a single cymbal beat on the fourth crotchet of bar 15. The therapist plays the two-beat pattern once again on the first two quavers of bar 16.

In the fourth phrase (bars 17–20) the melody contour is initially triadic in F major (bars 17–18) and leads stepwise downwards to the tonic in bars 18 and 19. This fourth phrase is followed by a three-bar pause. The therapist waits twice as long as between the first four phrases. During this time, the patient does not make any movement towards the cymbal with his foot.

Following this long pause, the therapist plays two short, melodically compact phrases (bars 24–28) at a lower dynamic level and with a steady slowing, or ritardando. This fifth phrase is a form of coda, emphasizing the closed symmetrical structure of the previous phrases. In this coda, the therapist sings 'we can play, we can play;' (original in German: 'wir können spielen, wir können spielen') on two tones and the episode closes on a chord of D major, the dominant chord of G major.

Summary of the four episodes of Bert's therapy (Episodes 1–4)

The four episodes (1–4) have been selected from Bert's music therapy. At the time of referral to music therapy Bert's foot movements were assessed by Bert's physiotherapist, occupational therapist and nurses as holding no communicative potential.

In the analysis of Episode 1 we see a possible synchronization between his foot movements and the music played by the therapist. Maybe the patient is synchronizing his foot movements to the music improvised by the therapist. This observation challenges the interpretation of his foot movements as meaningless, and demands a change in the assessment of Bert's perceptive and cognitive ability.

This is an exciting discovery. Bert's foot movements are potentially meaningful. At this time, this is also the only apparent possibility of experiencing contact with Bert. More significantly, it may be one of the only ways Bert can involve others in *his* activities. It is legitimate then to understand Bert's actions in terms of communication as opposed to uncontrolled reflexes.

Communication is a two-way street. Whether patients demonstrate communicative potential is dependent on their environment and we are that environment. It may be possible for a therapist to perceive subtle communicative acts if he or she is involved in an interactive communicative activity. The therapist will be led to this understanding only if he or she aims at creating a meaningful context that makes sense in terms of the patient's actions. Communication requires the interpretation of actions as being potentially communicative.

Events are described in Episode 2 in terms of their temporal context. A temporal context provides meaning between occurring events. If the patient and therapist's actions are ordered in a temporal context they may have a relational meaning. After moving in a 'sensible' moment in Episode 1, Bert's foot movement becomes embedded in a series of melodies in Episode 2. The therapist repeats the same melody referred to as 'A' in the analysis, each time Bert moves his foot. The participants begin to share a mutual understanding of this order of events. For a melody to be remembered by the patient, the therapist must play something memorable. This implies repetition and the recognition of sameness. Recognition of a melody is made simpler if it occurs at the same position in the order of repeating events.

The therapist changes his perception of the meaning of Bert's foot movements. As a result he is involved in a wider variety of Bert's movements, becoming increasingly aware of Bert's ability. He is not confined to testing the hypothetical 'meaninglessness' suggested before Bert's referral to music therapy.

The events in Episode 2 lead the therapist to believe in a potential 'de-isolation' of the patient. This change remedies a false isolation based on the seemingly perceptive restrictions shown by Bert. It may be that in situations of 'minimal' contact we search for gross signs of cognitive ability and miss those minute communicative signals and gestures from our patients. In this situation Bert actually changes because of how he is perceived. We may ask whether the patient has been attempting this communication earlier, but has been missing the necessary context or partner for communication. As Aldridge (2005) writes, we may have to consider calling these dialogical degenerative diseases where communication breaks down and we share answerability.

The therapist describes his own actions as *being directive* and Bert's actions as being *isolated actions*. Both of these constructs relate to the manner in which the therapist understands the communication. In this case the therapist is giving meaning to the actions of both participants. The therapist is trying to understand the communication. In this dialogue the patient attempts to recognize this understanding and to act in a perceived coordinated manner. The therapist is *being led* to understand the situation by the patient. Recognition in this sense is bringing events back into cognition.

By Episode 3 the therapist is more certain in his belief in Bert's recognition of patterns of interaction. Though the therapist is impelled to reinforce this sense of understanding by touching Bert's foot, it is the occasion on which Bert does not play that is the most significant event in this episode. At moments like this it is possible for the patient to exert **agency** and the therapist can release his control over the situation. This tells us much about the therapist's relationship with the patient. Through this the patient is empowered in his individuality, and can determine the course of not only his actions, but those of the therapist and the shared interaction.

In most settings patients with minute movement range are severely, if not completely, limited in realizing power and control over their activities. Bert begins to reduce this limitation. He conveys his need for communication. He is able to determine and participate in joint musical activities. The final episode (Episode 4, 'Foot cymbal') highlights the changes that have taken place in therapy in terms of **agency** and **motility**. In this episode, there is a revelation of Bert's ability to communicate musical content. As Bert initiates the two-bar pattern at the beginning of bar 4 in Episode 4, he demonstrates his recognition of musical exchange. He has begun to create structured musical material.

The positive change can be identified in the principal components analysis (please refer to Figure 3.2). The first three episodes appear close together in the bottom left quadrant, near to the constructs *being led, being directive, isolated actions, making sounds* and *questionable*. In contrast the fourth episode appears closer to the constructs *harmonic complexity, complex timbre, initiating* and *leading*.

The immense pressure caused by the possibly catastrophic psychological and cognitive isolation of a member of society begins to be lifted. Bert starts that process of recovery by which he will regain his situation in society. He is no longer without power or meaningful movement but has regained agency in some aspects of his life.

CHAPTER 5

Neil's Story: From Distress and Agitation to Humour and Joy – The Creation of a Dialogue

Neil and a bus collided. He was a normal healthy nine-year-old. A helicopter flew him to hospital where he was diagnosed with severe traumatic brain injury and required assisted breathing. At the time of admission to the rehabilitation clinic it was impossible to examine Neil's cognitive ability as he was continuously crying and screaming intensively. He followed movement of people and objects with his eyes. He had a right-side accented flexion in the upper limbs and left-side accented extension of the lower extremities. His feet were in tip-foot spastic position. He presented extreme muscle extension and later severe muscle flexion of his arms.

Episode 5: 'Crying'

Neil was crying and wailing. His face was covered in tears, his nose was running and his face was red and blotchy from the physical exertion of crying. His body was tightened by the grip of extreme high muscle tone, leading to a distortion of his body shape and an inability to use his limbs. Sleep was his only island of calm. The staff nurse said that most of the time that Neil was awake he cried. The ward staff were distraught and the ward doctor referred the young patient to individual music therapy with the plea, 'Can you do anything with him?' Although it was never mentioned explicitly, music therapy was not only seen as an adjunctive therapy but also a respite for the ward staff from Neil's crying and wailing. Fortunately, the music therapy room was soundproofed and two floors below the ward.

The episode is taken from the first moments of the first therapy session. Neil sits in a wheelchair near to the piano. As the episode begins, the therapist puts percussion beaters back into the cupboard before he goes to sit at the piano.

The human voice is not restricted to tones used in tuned instrumental music, so we also use a graphical notation here to suggest the general characteristics of the contours of the patient's voice when singing and crying as a sonogram. The sonogram is an adjunct to the notational transcription, providing another insight into a musical interpretation of the events.

The principal components analysis (see Figure 3.2) shows Episode 5 near to the constructs *responding* (category **agency**), *distress* (category **emotionality**), *small utterance* (category **communication**) and *simple timbre* (category **musical expression**).

To analyse Episode 5 (Figure 5.1) a sonogram of the episode has been created (Figure 5.2). The sonogram image shows only frequencies below 1838 Hz.

At the beginning of the episode Neil is heard weeping and we then hear two very short tones ('f#3' and 'b3'), played by the therapist on the piano (0:00.09–0:00.10), followed by a chord consisting of 'b' and 'f#' (0:00.11) (see Figure 5.2). The third tone of the triad, 'd', is played later (0:00.14/bar 7) and makes the tonality of B minor explicit. The therapist is *responding* to the *small utterances* made by Neil by defining a tonal space for his vocalizations.

By viewing the sonogram we can uncover a relationship between Neil's weeping and the therapist's initial actions. The second tone 'f#', played by the therapist (0:00.10/bar 5, beat 3), matches the pitch of the first of Neil's vocalizations. The therapist is trying to find the tone that corresponds to the patient's vocalization. In combination with Neil's second vocalization (0:00.03–0:00.06/bar 3) that circles around the tone 'd4', the triad of tones belonging to the chord of B minor have been heard ('b', 'd' and 'f#').

Episode 5

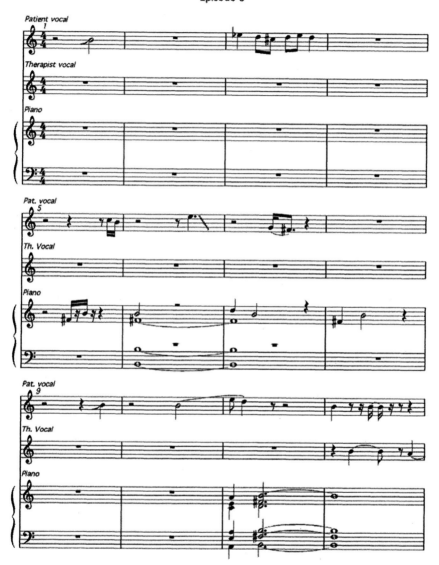

Figure 5.1 Transcription of Episode 5

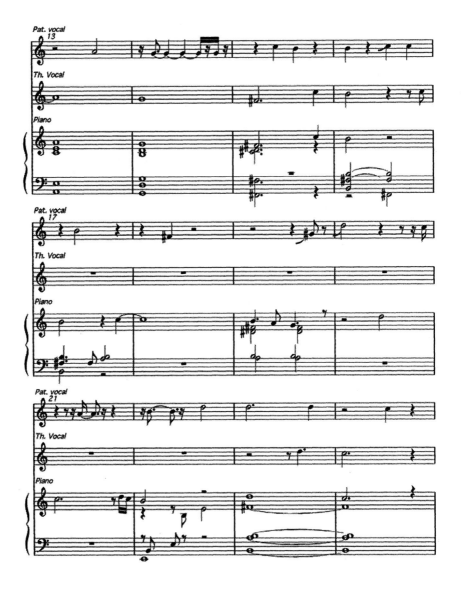

Figure 5.1 Transcription of Episode 5 (continued)

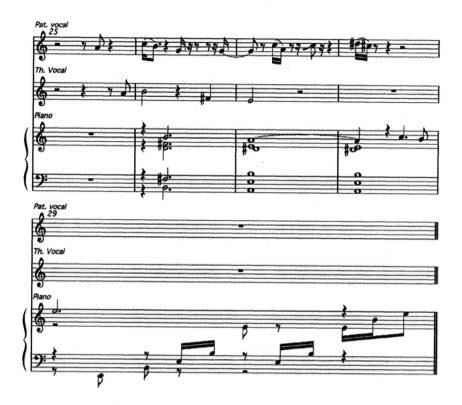

Figure 5.1 Transcription of Episode 5 (continued)

In this episode Neil is making *small utterances,* mostly single tones or single vocalizations as in bars 15–18. The therapist matches these tones in pitch. Neil and the therapist are *responding* to each other by imitating the pitch of each other's vocalizations and the pitches played on the piano (see grey squares in Figure 5.3).

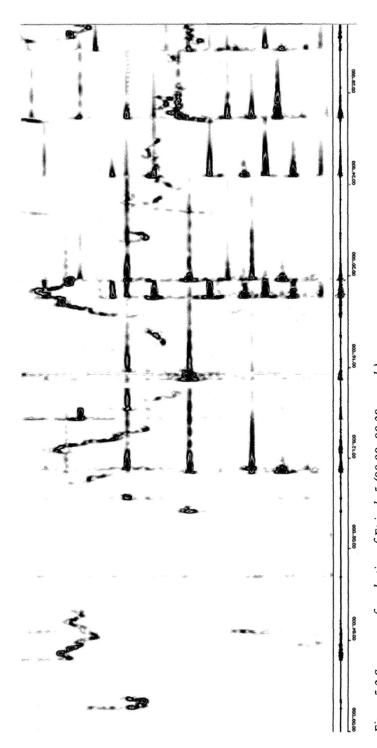

Figure 5.2 Sonogram of a selection of Episode 5 (00.00—00.29 seconds)

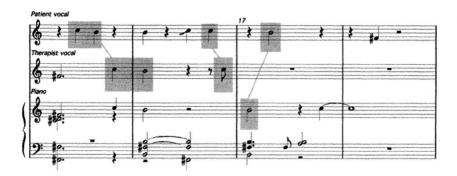

Figure 5.3 Bars 15–18 of Episode 5

In this excerpt Neil sings a two-tone ('c', 'b') falling motive in bar 15 on beats 2–3 that is directly mirrored by the therapist. At the end of bar 16 the therapist imitates the previous tone 'c' sung by Neil. At the beginning of bar 17 the therapist plays the tone 'b', which is then imitated by Neil on the second beat of the bar. Neil's vocalizations have a quality of *distress*. The tension created in his vocalizations between the minor ninth tone 'c' in the tonality of B minor and the tonic tone 'b' is mirrored in the vocalizations of the therapist. The tension caused by this harmony is experienced by the therapist as an expression of Neil's **emotionality**; with tears on his cheeks, the patient looks and sounds in *distress*.

In the transcription in Figure 5.4 we can see Neil leading the therapist in a downward series of tones in bars 20–22. On bar 22, beat 3, Neil then sings the minor third 'd' of the tonality. It is the therapist who leads the melody downwards on the tones 'd', 'c', 'a', 'b' and 'f#' and ends on the tone 'e' in bar 27. Neil does not follow this contour to the end, and in bar 27 moves upwards towards the tonic 'e' reaching only the tones 'd#' and 'c#'. In bar 29 the therapist releases the harmonic tension in bar 29, emphasizing a modulation to E minor in bar 21.

Neil's actions are fascinating in this episode. He is obviously in *distress*, his crying sounds like desperate calls from deep within. He is isolated. In the music improvisation, there are clear signs of a coordination between the pitches of Neil's music making and that of the therapist. That is what the therapist intends as a central technique in this approach. It is an attempt at inclusion, moving from isolation to inclusion. Music therapy provides a unique situation of participation. Distress is not

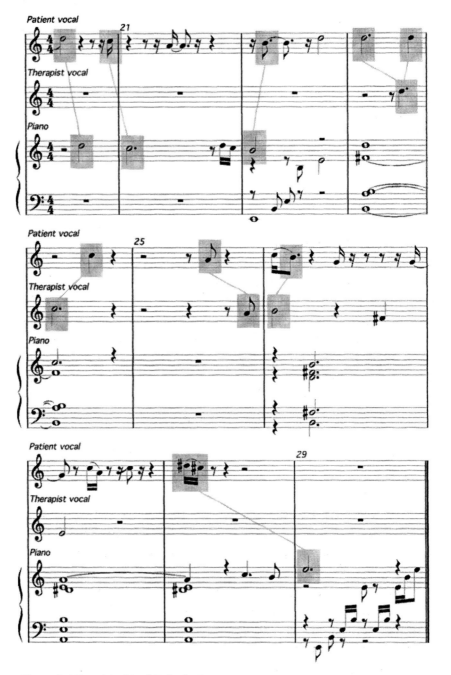

Figure 5.4 Bars 20–29 of Episode 5

negated, but from the expression of distress it is possible to mirror the sound component of that distress and, in musical expression, offer the possibility of moving from distress and isolation to another state.

Episode 6: 'Hello Neil'

This episode is taken from the second therapy session with Neil on 9 August 1994. Neil is vocalizing to the sound 'ah', and the therapist is playing the piano and singing with the simple greeting 'Hallo Neil'. The episode is 37 seconds in duration.

In the principal components analysis Episode 6 appears near to the constructs *harmonic simplicity* and *simple timbre*. Both these constructs are related to the category **musical expression**. The episode is also shown near to the construct *vocal*, which belongs to the category **motility**.

The tonality of the episode is F major, and though the therapist often uses a seventh chord (bar 2) and various inversions, the harmonic vocabulary is limited to three chords, B flat major seventh chord (see bars 2, 5, and 9), F major (bar 8) and D major (bar 11). The *harmonic simplicity* in the piano accompaniment reflects the *simple timbre* of the unaccompanied sections in which the patient sings alone. Both of these aspects belong to the category **musical expression**, and the episode demonstrates clear and simple musical material used in the interaction.

Neil vocalizes using pitches belonging to the tonality used by the therapist. His voice sounds like whining, not in pain, but has more of the character of *distress*. All his vocalizations lack pronunciation and are made to the sound 'ah'. The *simple timbre* of his voice is shallow, thin and baby-like. At the same time Neil is mirroring the melodic contours sung by the therapist. It appears as if he is trying to coordinate his singing with that of the therapist, whilst experiencing a contrasting mood.

In Episode 6 (Figure 5.5) Neil and therapist are exchanging short melodies, copying the tempo and melodic contour. In the excerpt from the transcription in Figure 5.6 we can see the therapist imitating melodies sung by the patient.

Episode 6: Hello Neil

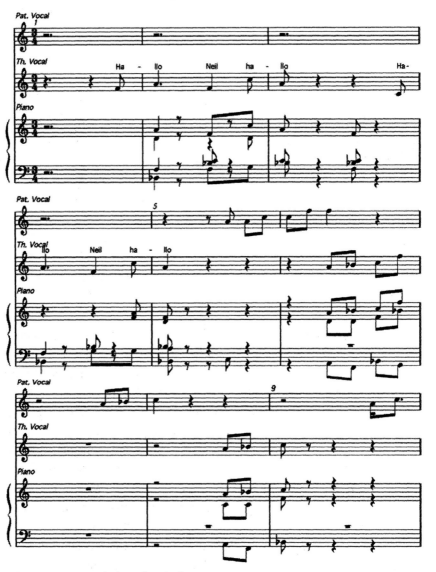

Figure 5.5 Transcription of Episode 6

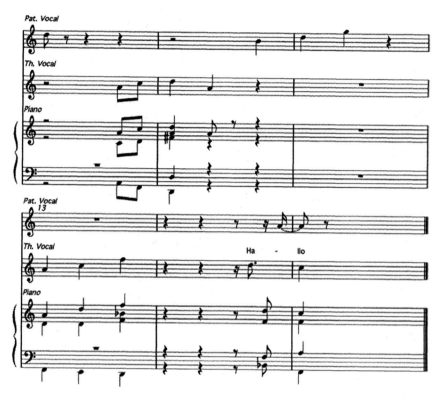

Figure 5.5 Transcription of Episode 6 (continued)

In this episode the patient's *vocal* expressions are becoming more tonally related to the music made by the therapist. The vocalizations have taken on the form of short phrases, as opposed to a collection of single tones. These phrases have a wider range and Neil's voice shows more **motility** than in Episode 5. We can infer from this that there is an intention on the part of Neil to actively participate. He has a role to play in his recovery by forming his reponses and actively evoking responses from his therapist, which is surely the basis of communication.

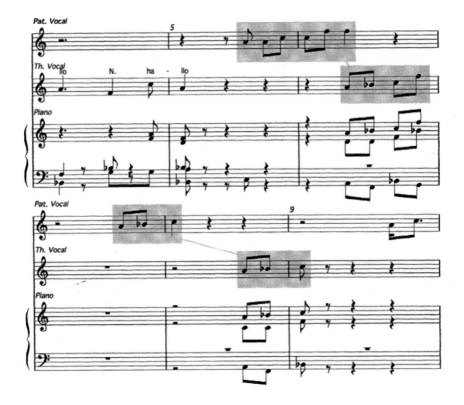

Figure 5.6 Bars 4–9 of Episode 6

Episode 7: 'From behind the covers'

The therapist sings, 'Hello Neil, we can sing.' Neil sings very soft, separate tones in reply and the therapist accompanies on the piano.

Episode 7 (Figure 5.7) appears near to the constructs *vocal* (category **motility**) and *harmonic simplicity* (category **musical expression**) in the principal components analysis.

The patient's vocalizations are quiet, short, whimper-like sounds. The therapist sings gently to the text 'Hello Neil, we can sing' (original text: 'Hallo Neil, wir können singen') at the beginning of the episode. The tonality of the improvisation is F major and the patient vocalizes on either the tonic tone 'f' or on the tones 'e', 'd' and 'g'. The accompaniment to the patient's *vocal* sounds is sparse, and controlled with *harmonic simplicity*, and matches the tones sung by the patient with single tones at times (Figure 5.8).

Episode 7: From behind the covers

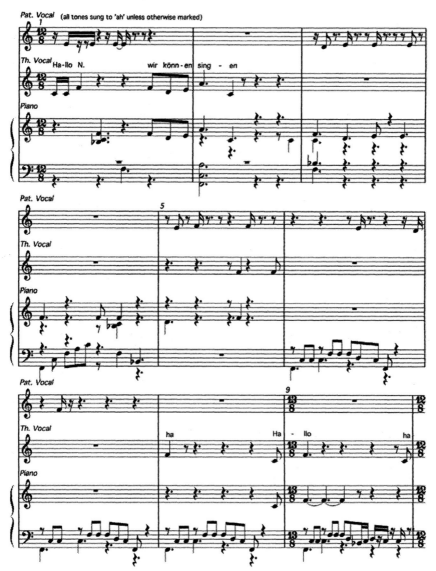

Figure 5.7 Transcription of Episode 7

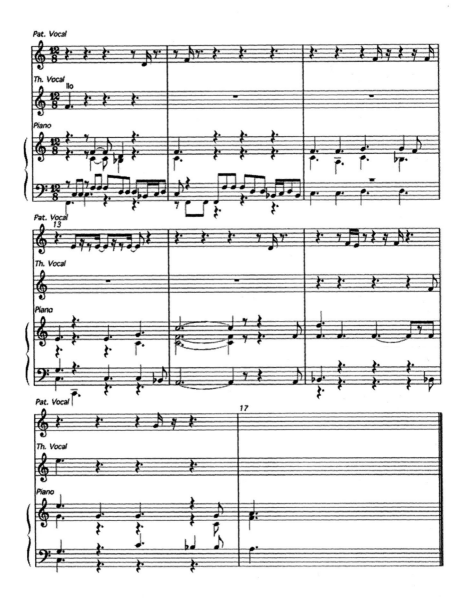

Figure 5.7 Transcription of Episode 7 (continued)

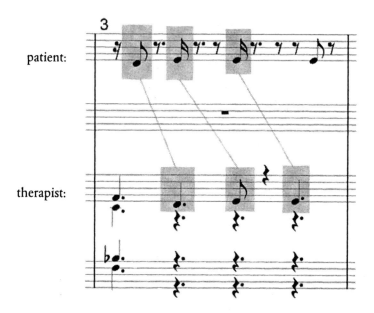

Figure 5.8 Bar 3 of Episode 7

The patient also matches the pitches played on the piano by the therapist (Figure 5.9).

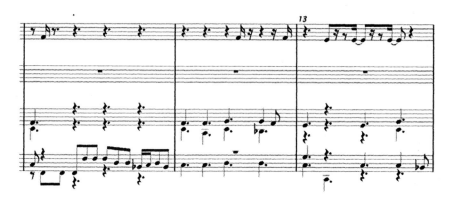

Figure 5.9 Bars 11–13 of Episode 7

In bar 11 we can see the patient vocalizing on the tone 'f', shortly after the therapist plays the same tone on the piano. Later, in bar 12, the patient imitates the tone 'f' played previously by the therapist twice. In the following bar the patient once again imitates the tone 'e' played on the piano by the therapist. The patient and therapist are involved in direct imitation.

The patient's voice sounds timid and tentative. It is very quiet and sounds as though he is experimenting in controlling his breath and voice. The therapist creates a balance between mirroring this tentativeness through playing single tones on the piano (bars 3 and 5) with phrases of light, playful motives in the bass accompaniment (bars 6–11) (Figure 5.10).

The increased level of motion in the bass accompaniment tends towards change away from the tentative and introspective quality of Neil's vocalizations. Using these musical suggestions, maintaining the temporal and harmonic space through the episode, we can integrate Neil's expressions. Thus the therapist both mirrors the sounds that Neil makes, and also makes suggestions for possible musical development within a coherent harmonic and temporal context. It is here that we see

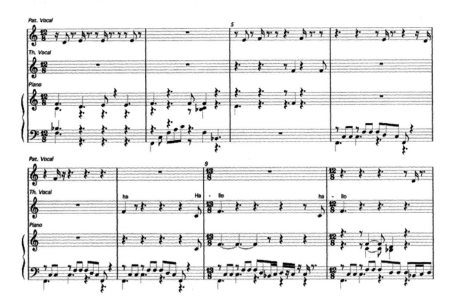

Figure 5.10 Bars 3–10 of Episode 7

how sounds become music by offering Neil's utterances a rich context for development. The activity of sounding in time is interactive. These sounds make sense in all the various interpretations of sense-making. They gain meaning in terms of interaction in the communication between the therapist and Neil, in an external sense. But internally, we can speculate that Neil is integrating his vocal capabilities with his aural and cognitive capabilities.

Episode 8: 'Hello Simon'

One week has passed since the session from which Episode 7 was taken. Neil and the therapist are playing around and alternating greetings by singing 'Hallo Neil' and 'Hallo Simon'. The mood is playful and the piano accompaniment reminds of the vamping style of pantomime theatre music. At the end of the episode, the therapist starts off a word-completion game using the text 'hal…llo'.

Episode 8 (Figure 5.11) appears near to the constructs *occurs in and out* and *conventional use of instrument* in the principal components analysis. It appears in the quadrant that includes the constructs *leading* and *non-directive*.

The construct *occurs in and out* belongs to the category **participation**. The *conventional use of instrument* belongs to the category **motility**. The construct *leading* belongs to the category **agency**, and the construct *non-directive* is found in the category **communication**.

In this episode Neil greets the therapist by saying 'Hallo Simon'. This is the first time the therapist has heard the patient speaking since the beginning of the rehabilitation process and is something that now *occurs in and out* of the music therapy setting. The greeting song that follows is characterized by playful exchanges. By regaining the ability to speak and sing selected words the patient is able to **participate** in vocal and verbal interaction.

Neil is 'playing around'. We can hear this in his strong and clear voice and his hearty laughter. His voice sounds more *conventional*, fitting to a boy of his age. His vocalizations are flexible and his voice shows signs of more **motility**.

Neil is playing a game in an improvised song with the therapist. He is playing around with his name and that of the therapist. At some points he

Episode 8: Hallo Simon

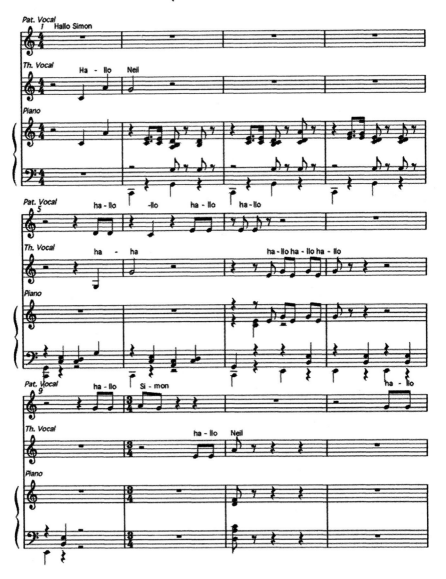

Figure 5.11 Transcription of Episode 8

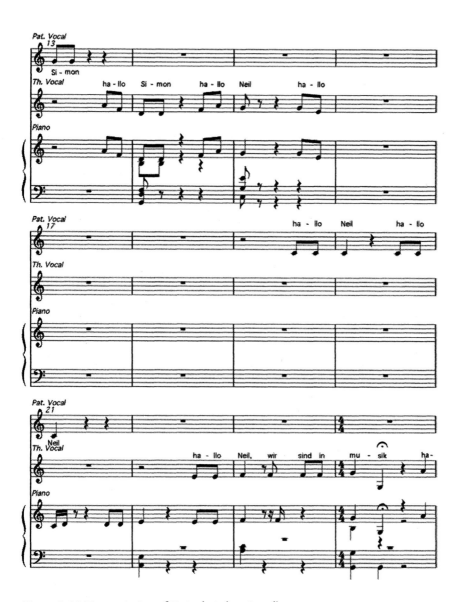

Figure 5.11 Transcription of Episode 8 (continued)

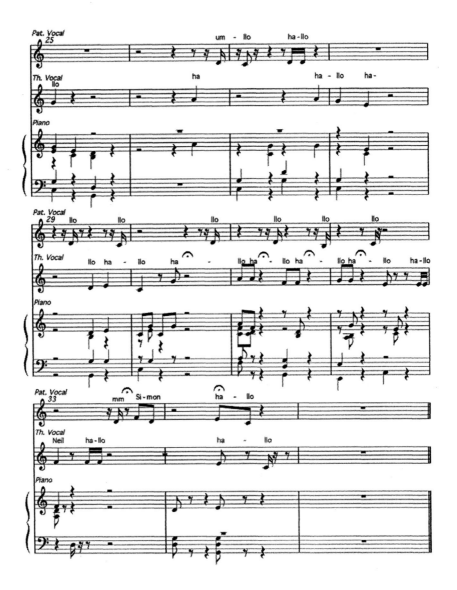

Figure 5.11 Transcription of Episode 8 (continued)

exchanges his name with that of the therapist and 'breaks' the rules of greetings. Neil obviously finds it funny that the therapist 'plays along' in switching names. He is recognizing humour and playing with the organization of patterns of social interaction.

The therapist leaves large pauses in which Neil can *lead* the improvised song. Combined with his relaxed and humorous mood, the level of **agency** he has in this episode is high. He is able to determine the course of interaction (Figure 5.12).

Following a short pause in bar 24 the therapist involves Neil in a 'word completion' passage (bars 26–34). The 'game' for the patient is to complete the first half of the word 'hallo' sung by the therapist (Figure 5.13).

We can see in bars 26, 29, 30 and 31 the patient completing the word 'hallo' with very short 'llos'. This passage is made up of sequenced phrases that begin on the fifth quaver of bar 30 and end on the fifth quaver of bar 32. Neil's vocalizations are quieter than in the rest of the episode, but sound determined and vocally focused. He sounds like a little boy, and not like a fearful baby as in earlier episodes. He appears to be confident and focused in the interaction. He is **participating** in the duet as a singer, *leading* parts of the improvisation, and is offered improvised suggestions from the therapist that are *non-directive*.

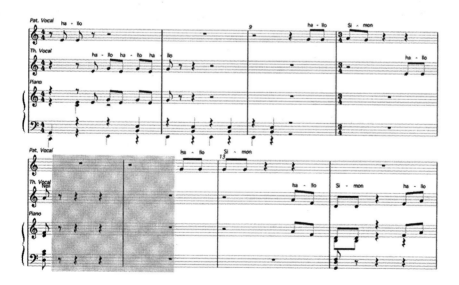

Figure 5.12 Bars 7–14 of Episode 8

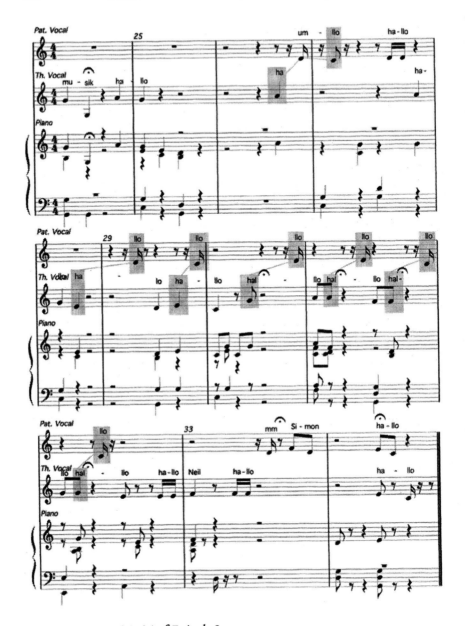

Figure 5.13 Bars 24–34 of Episode 8

Summary of Episodes 5–8 selected from music therapy with Neil

Neil was referred to music therapy specifically to attempt at providing a means of entering into contact. Floods of tears accompanied his crying and wailing. He was obviously in distress and showed no means of expressing himself verbally. As Aldridge (2001, p.14) has pointed out, 'Agitation in children is a communication and attempts to provide the child with comfort, support, and alternative ways to communicate help.' Therefore it was necessary to understand Neil, not in terms of words, but through the actions and sounds he was producing. The therapist focused on the musical qualities of his vocalizations. In the early sessions he concentrated on matching the pitch and melodic contours of Neil's vocal expressions. As seen in the analysis of Episodes 5, 6 and 7, Neil increasingly *responded* with vocal exchanges and began tonally imitating the music played by the therapist on the piano. His initial *small utterances* were embedded in a flowing musical structure. Later he began imitating and initiating musical exchanges.

In these three episodes (5, 6 and 7), a change takes place in the meaning of Neil's vocalizations from crying to singing. Once interpreted as 'singing', it is possible to concentrate on the variation of musical parameters that Neil uses in his vocalizations. These elements of musical expression are the stuff of communication in music therapy. In the analysis we have seen that it is not simply the fact that Neil increases his range of musical expression that determines positive change but that he has, together with the therapist, been able to be musically communicative and to experience interaction. It is this experience of interaction that is clinically significant. Within this interaction it is possible for Neil to develop a repertoire of communication that may later be transferred to settings outside of music therapy.

It is essential that changes within a therapy situation be transferable to other situations in the patient's life. This transfer relates to the relevance of therapeutic change for the patient in rehabilitation. If the patient is able to make use of his experiences in a therapy setting in other situations in his or her life, we may speak of success in therapy.

In the final episode selected from therapy with Neil, we have seen him begin using his singing in a game about social interaction. The musical interaction observed in earlier episodes and his repertoire of musical expressivity remains apparent in his vocal expression. Most importantly, Neil has been able to take control. He determines the length of pauses and the course of interaction. The therapist's actions are *non-directive* and Neil is *leading* the improvisation. Most significant for Neil's overall rehabilitation is his change in mood. Neil is no longer in *distress* and is much *calm*er. This change is not only important for music therapy, but for Neil's whole rehabilitation process. He is able to concentrate on events occurring in his environment and is not so psychologically introverted as at the outset. He has become able to imitate his communication partners and begin to relearn important processes.

It is also important at this stage in his recovery that Neil can experience fun. He is nine years old, and will be challenged by the consequences of his traumatic brain injury in the future. Positive life experiences at this stage in his life will enhance his future development. For his family, laughter and joy means more than an external observer can assess. After many weeks of distress and crying, the whole family will enjoy such moments of happiness. Neil laughs in the music therapy and also at home.

CHAPTER 6

Mark's Story: A Fusion of Two Worlds – Physical Dependency and Creative Partnership

Mark was born in 1968 and is a qualified motor mechanic who worked in a garage repairing haulage trucks. In July 1998 he had a severe motorcycle accident. Mark lost control of his motorcycle on quiet country road, collided with a barrier and was thrown into the adjacent field. He was found by chance, at the site of the accident, by a passing doctor. Unconscious, without blood pressure or pulse, it was necessary to give him mouth-to-mouth respiration and external heart massage. Following extensive diagnostic procedures, he was found to have severe traumatic brain injury, a severely broken hip, multiple bruising and various skin abrasions. Because of the brain injury he suffered, he was initially paralysed from his neck downwards.

Following emergency treatment and intensive care, Mark was admitted for early neurosurgical rehabilitation. He presented tetraparesis,[1] facial nerve dysfunction, a reduction of the choke reflex, and an extreme increase of flexion of both hands. He could not move, he could not speak and was not able to make any vocal sounds.

Mark began individual music therapy in September of the same year.

---

1   Muscular weakness of all four limbs.

Episode 9: 'Light in a dark night'

Episode 9 originates from a session eight months after his accident and has been selected from one of the first improvisations in which Mark played a MIDI synthesizer (Yamaha).

In the episode, Mark is playing the synthesizer with his left hand using an input device specifically designed and built for him by the therapist. This device consists of a photoelectric cell that reacts to different amounts of light emitted from a small hand torch reflected from a wooden board placed at an angle to the sensor. The pitch of the synthesizer is determined by the amount of light registered by the photoelectric cell. This device enables Mark to play a two-octave range of notes with the sound of a synthesized flute with a minimum of physical movement. Mark was only able to move his wrist 2–3 centimetres at this time. The restriction of the device means that the user can only play neighbouring tones, the dynamic and duration are pre-defined, and each tone is released once a new tone is played. Any leaps between tones result from an error in the synthesizer signal processing. The therapist accompanies Mark on the piano and the improvisation is in a light pop-ballad style.

Episode 9 (Figure 6.1) appears near to the constructs *complex timbre* (category **musical expression**), *initiating* (category **agency**) and *calm* (category **emotionality**) in the principal components analysis.

In the episode, Mark is playing a keyboard that produces a synthesized sound similar to that of two flutes playing simultaneously. In combination with the sound of the acoustic piano, this produces a *complex timbre*. By choosing the synthesized flute sound, Mark makes a decision about his **musical expression**.

In Figure 6.2 we can see a representation of the amplitudes of the recording of the episode under the grey time code bar. In the middle block we see a graphic representation of the pitches played by Mark. The lowest element in the graphic shows a representation of the transcription of the tones played by the therapist on the piano. A prominent form, obvious in the overview of the episode transcription, is the light semi-circular curve of the melody line played by the patient.

The patient takes *initiative* in creating the melodic form of the improvisation. We can see rising and falling phrases spiralling in an upward direction in the short excerpt in Figure 6.3.

Episode 9: Light in a dark night

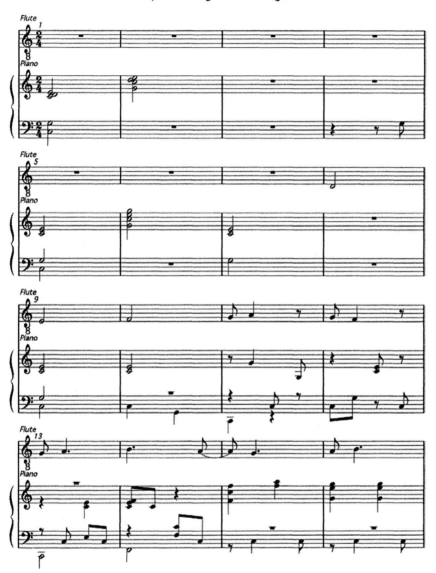

Figure 6.1 Transcription of Episode 9

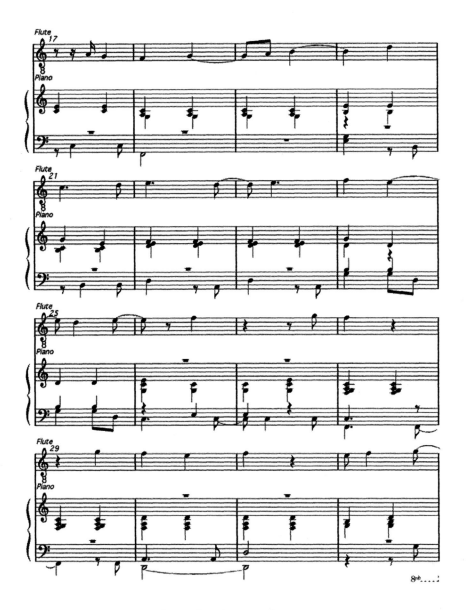

Figure 6.1 Transcription of Episode 9 (continued)

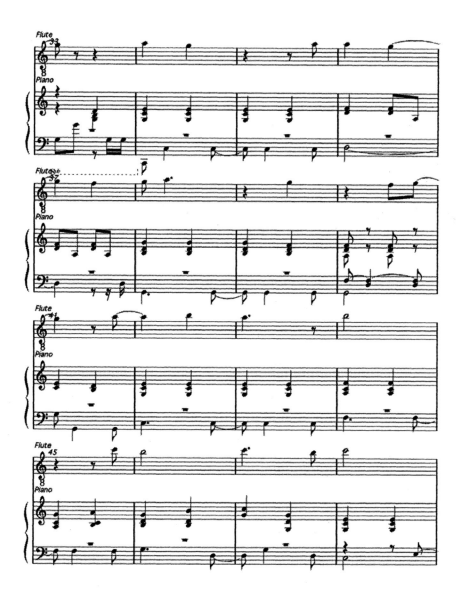

Figure 6.1 Transcription of Episode 9 (continued)

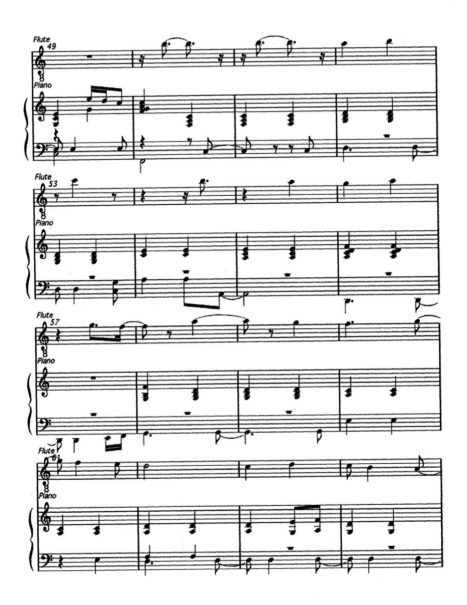

Figure 6.1 Transcription of Episode 9 (continued)

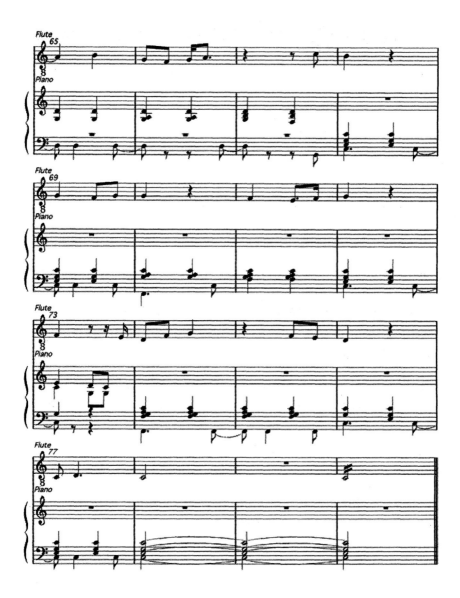

Figure 6.1 Transcription of Episode 9 (continued)

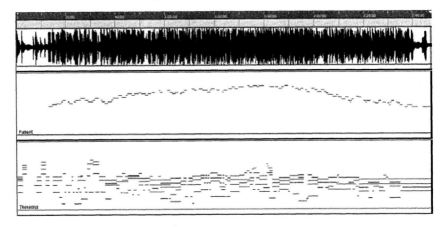

Figure 6.2 Overview of Episode 9

Mark's melody reaches a climax on the tone 'c' in bar 48 accompanied by a cadence in C major on the piano. This tone is the highest tone that can be played on the synthesized instrument. Following this climax we hear a slow, stepwise downward movement over two octaves before the improvisation comes to a close.

This episode is taken from the second occasion on which Mark was able to play using a two-octave range of tones, made possible by an input device for a MIDI synthesizer that required only a minimal range of movement. This allowed Mark to *lead* the improvisation and to be an **agent** of the course of events. Mark's melodic improvising also determined the harmonic structure of the improvisation and led the therapist's piano playing (Figure 6.4).

In bar 25 Mark moves from the tone 'e' to the tone 'f' on the second beat of the bar. Though the therapist does not immediately react to this change, remaining in the harmonic phrasing, he is led to choosing to play the chord of F major in bar 28. In bar 29 there is a further example of Mark leading the therapist's improvising. Mark begins a melodic phrase on the tone 'g' and the therapist expects him to play either the neighbour tone 'f' or 'a'. In accord with the two-bar harmonic phrasing, a chord change is to be expected in bar 30. The therapist chooses to play a D minor chord, in which both the tones 'f' and 'a' are found. Therefore, the therapist is being *led* in his choice of harmony by Mark.

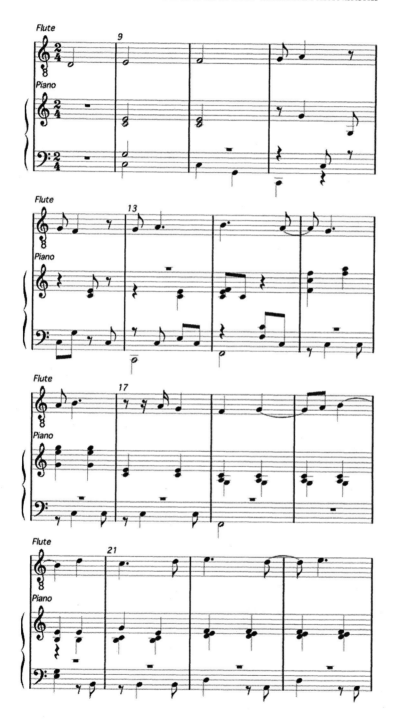

Figure 6.3 Bars 8–23 of Episode 9

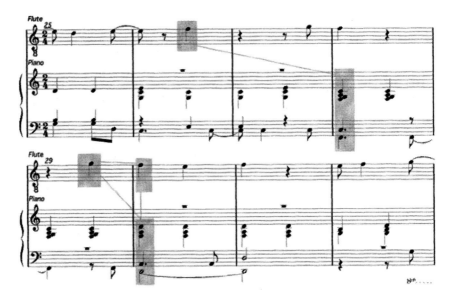

Figure 6.4 Bars 25–32 of Episode 9

Mark's instrument is restricted to producing neighbouring tones of the C major scale ranging from 'c3' to 'c5'. This limits the choice of tones that can be played. There are occasions in which interval leaps can be heard (bars 20, 58, 65–66, 66–67, 68–69 and 74). This is because of an inconsistency in the generation of sounds by the synthesizer.

The curved form of the melody, with a thematic climax at approximately two-thirds of the episode, and the harmonic accompaniment, lends a sense of *calm*ness to the episode. In addition, the synthesizer sound chosen by the patient is warm and sonorous. These aspects characterize the **emotionality** of the episode.

Episode 10: 'The flute is my voice'

Episode 10 is taken from the music therapy session with Mark one month later. Mark is playing a synthesizer with a small touch-sensitive MIDI keyboard with three-octave range. He plays with the extended index finger of his left hand, which is clenched in a fist with a high level of flexion in his wrist. As in Episode 9 Mark selected a synthesized flute sound; the therapist also plays a synthesizer and uses a synthesized orchestral sound.

The transcription of Episode 10 (Figure 6.5) is without bar-lines. The rhythmic values of the tones are presented reflecting a sense of pulse as opposed to a metrical value. The transcription focuses on the harmonic and melodic aspects of the episode.

In the principal components analysis, Episode 10 appears near to the constructs *instrumental* (category **motility**) and *complex timbre* and *harmonic complexity* (category **musical expression**).

The music is *instrumental*; Mark and the therapist are both playing synthesizers via keyboards. Mark plays a synthesized sound of two flutes. The therapist uses a sound of multiple synthesized stringed instruments. These instruments are characterized by a *complex timbre*. Each sound consists of a combination of multiple synthesized instruments.

Mark is playing a synthesizer with his hand using a small MIDI keyboard. Since Episode 9 his range of movement has increased and he is able to move his hand with movements of his lower arm from the elbow. The keyboard facilitates dynamic expression in the duration and loudness of each tone. The attack of each note reacts to the velocity of the movement of the keys. If the key is struck more firmly, the attack of the sound is pronounced. In contrast, if the key is pressed lightly, the attack is reduced and the sound will build up more slowly. The increase in Mark's **motility** enables him to reach a higher level of **musical expression**.

The *complex timbre* of the instruments in Episode 10, together with the *harmonic complexity* of the improvisation, determines the intensity of **musical expression**. Complex chords, including minor seventh chords (fifth beat of the first system), and minor chords with added intervals of the sixth and seventh (second crotchet beat of system 4) played by the therapist, are examples of harmonic complexity.

In the episode there are complex harmonic structures that result from the intertwining music played by Mark and the therapist. One example is the progression seen in system 7. The therapist plays a octave interval of the tone 'a', with a ninth interval ('b'), and Mark adds the tone 'e' to create an implicit chord in the tonality of 'a', which omits an explicit sounding of the third of the scale. This omission makes the tonality of the chord unclear.

Episode 10: The flute is my voice

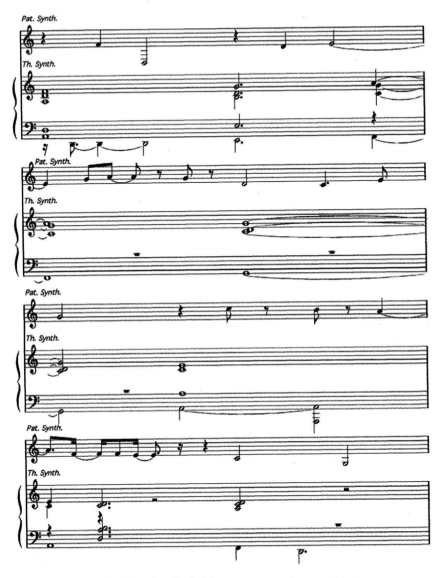

Figure 6.5 Transcription of Episode 10

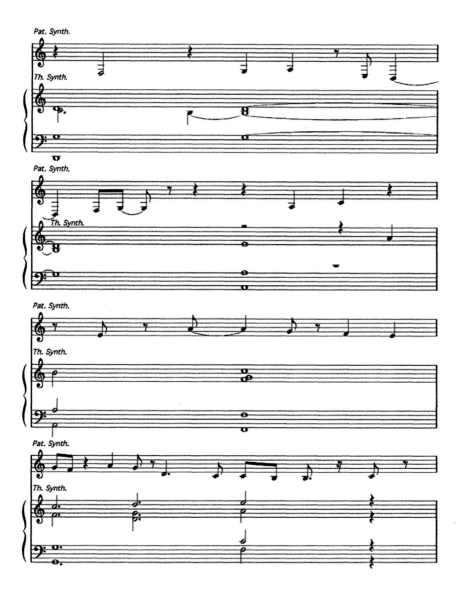

Figure 6.5 Transcription of Episode 10 (continued)

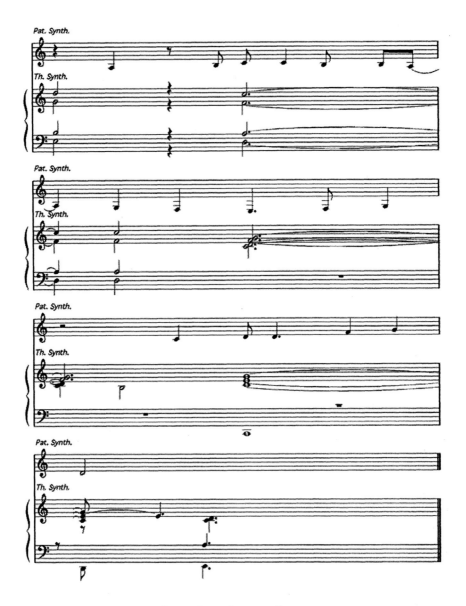

Figure 6.5 Transcription of Episode 10 (continued)

The therapist is using a range of harmonic vocabulary. This vocabulary includes altered chords, triadic chords with additional tones. These chords come about through the combination of the tones played by Mark and the therapist. In other situations, the therapist uses clusters of tones as in the middle of system 10. In systems 8 and 9 the therapist improvises a sequential chord passage. The chords used by the therapist are triadic chords with addition intervals of a seventh (Figure 6.6).

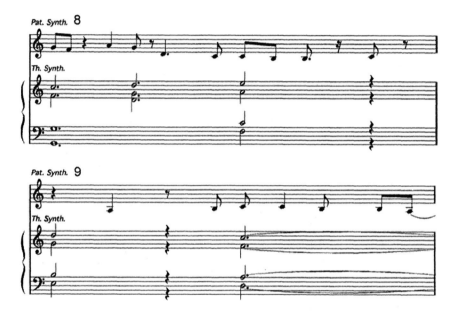

Figure 6.6 System 8 and 9 of Episode 9

The mood of the music improvised in Episode 10 is ambiguous. The harmonic changes between major and relative minor chords give a sense of changeability. There is a sense of serenity in the music, though a quality of sorrow can also be heard. These interpretations do not mean that the music is serene or sorrowful, but that the music evokes a feeling of serenity and sorrow.

Episode 11: 'Steel drum'

In Episode 11 Mark is heard alone playing a Caribbean steel drum (Figure 6.7). The steel drum is tuned using a five-tone, or pentatonic, scale beginning on the tone 'f'. The episode is selected from a therapy session that took place in August of the same year. The therapist is sitting by the side of Mark, and takes part as an active listener.

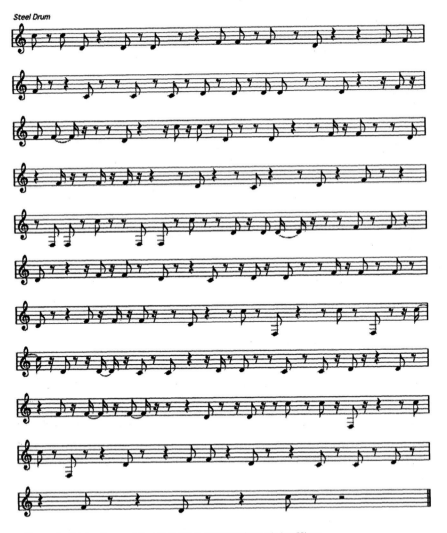

Episode 11: Steel drum

Please note: Note lengths are relative values, tempo of quantised transcription=55bpm

Figure 6.7 Transcription of Episode 11

The transcription of Episode 11 is without bar-lines. The rhythmic values of the tones are presented reflecting a sense of pulse as opposed to a metrical value. The note lengths are related to relative values and the quantization of the transcription was carried out at 55 beats per minute. The transcription focuses on the melodic aspects of the episode.

Episode 11 appears near to the constructs *non-directive, making music* and *integrated actions* in the principal components analysis. These constructs belong to the category **communication**.

The therapeutic intervention in the episode is *non-directive*. The therapist participates as an active listener and Mark is playing the steel drum alone.

It is clear that Mark is *making music*, as opposed to experimenting with sounds, or simply making sounds. This is apparent in the coherent phrasing and repetition of melodic patterns in his playing. The example in Figure 6.8 highlights the organization and repetition of a melodic pattern. The melodic cell 'f–f–f–d' is marked with grey shading.

These cells are part of large melodic structures, which can be heard as *leitmotif*, returning after short passages of thematic variation. The two motives in this episode are marked in Figure 6.9 as 'A' and 'B' and repetitions are numbered.

The phrases played by Mark are *integrated actions*. His improvisation is *calm* and tranquil. The dynamic is at a moderate level and the timbre of the steel drum adds to a sense of mysticism and serenity. Though there is no metrical division of passing time, the episode does not lack cohesion. This cohesion may stem from a temporal variation in the presentation of the various melodic motives.

There is also a balance between Mark's use of large intervallic leaps, shown in grey squares in Figure 6.10, and neighbouring tones (of the pentatonic scale), shown in grey ellipses. The excerpt is taken from the end of the episode.

Episode 12: '9th September'

Episode 12 is taken from a music therapy session with Mark that took place one month later, in September. Mark plays a three-octave chromatic metallophone with a soft beater and the therapist plays the piano. In addition to these two instruments a drum machine was also used. The

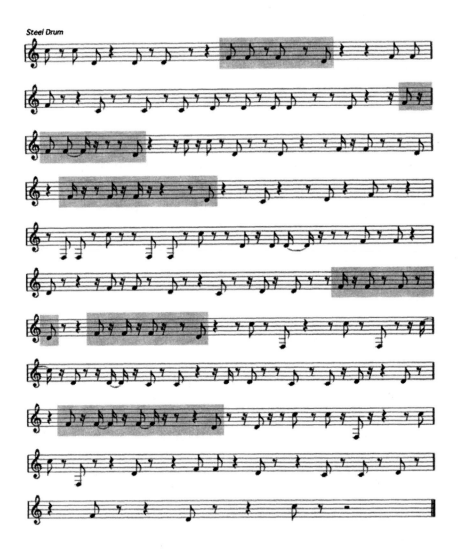

Figure 6.8 Repetition of melodic patterns in Episode 11

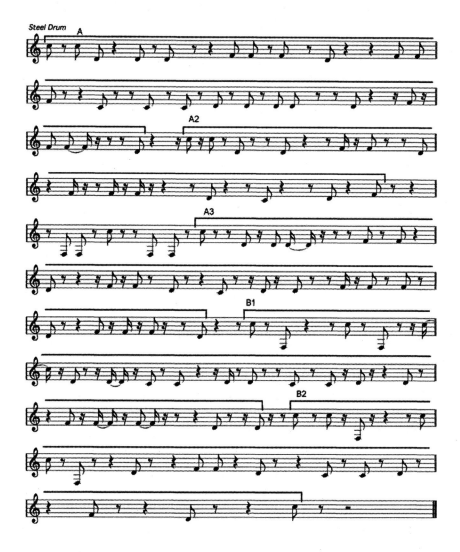

Figure 6.9 Phrase structures in Episode 11

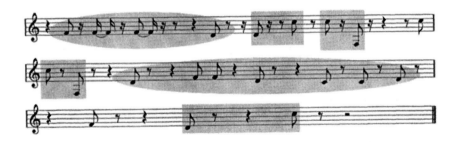

Figure 6.10 Use of intervallic leaps and neighbouring tones in Episode 11

rhythmic pattern was designed by Mark and programmed by the therapist. The episode is 2 minutes 27 seconds in duration.

Figure 6.11 shows the signs used in the music transcription of Episode 12.

Drum machine:

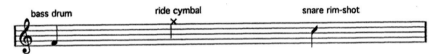

Figure 6.11 Signs used in the transcription of Episode 12

Episode 12 (Figure 6.12) appears near to the constructs *extended play, certainty* and *making music* (category **communication**) and the construct *initiating* (category **agency**) in the principal components analysis.

A drum machine plays a cool, lightly swung pattern that Mark designed. The drum machine plays two bars alone before Mark *initiates* the first phrase. This melodic phrase is finely syncopated, arriving at each tone slightly earlier than the metronomic drums. This syncopation reflects the swing-style syncopated bass drum beat heard shortly before the third beat and the snare drum rim-shot beats heard shortly before the fourth beat of each bar. The drum machine provides Mark and therapist with a temporal orientation to coordinate their improvising. The episode is taken from a therapy session in which the therapist was *certain* of the patient's intentions and wishes. Mark and the therapist had discussed the instrumentation and drum pattern before the improvisation began.

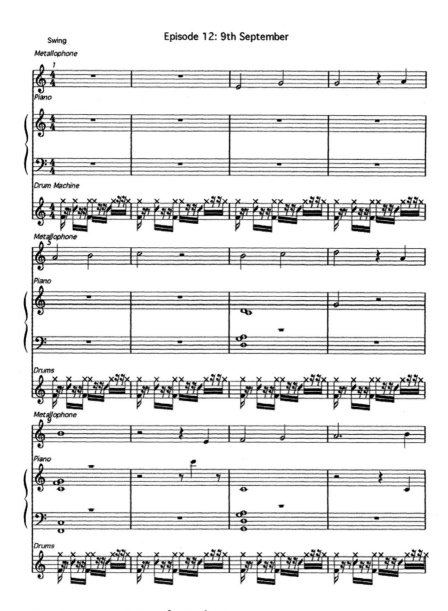

Figure 6.12 Transcription of Episode 12

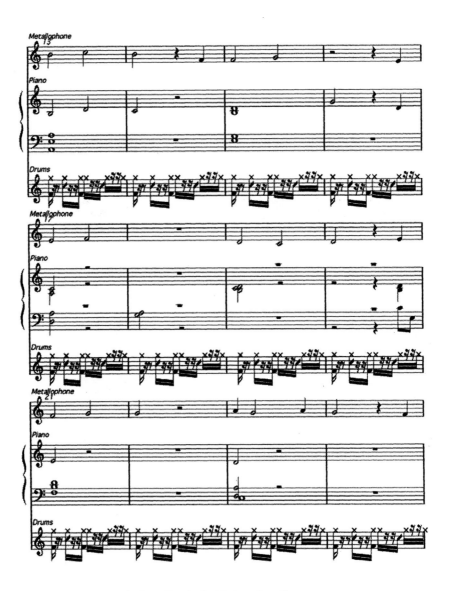

Figure 6.12 Transcription of Episode 12 (continued)

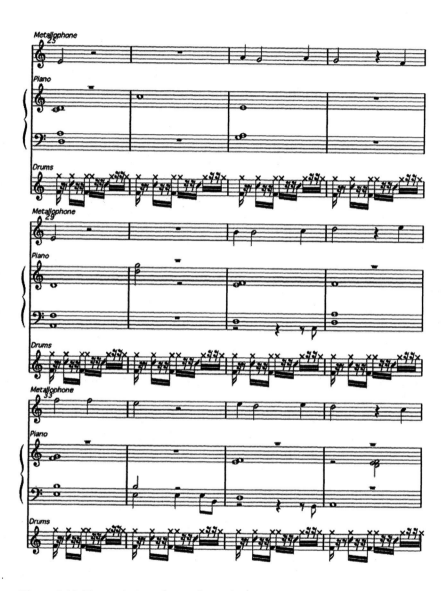

Figure 6.12 Transcription of Episode 12 (continued)

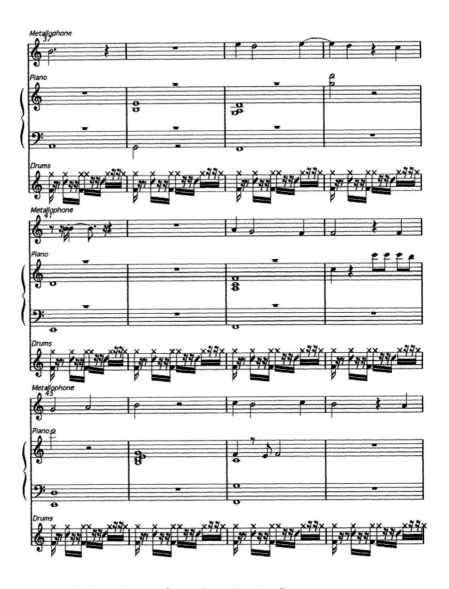

Figure 6.12 Transcription of Episode 12 (continued)

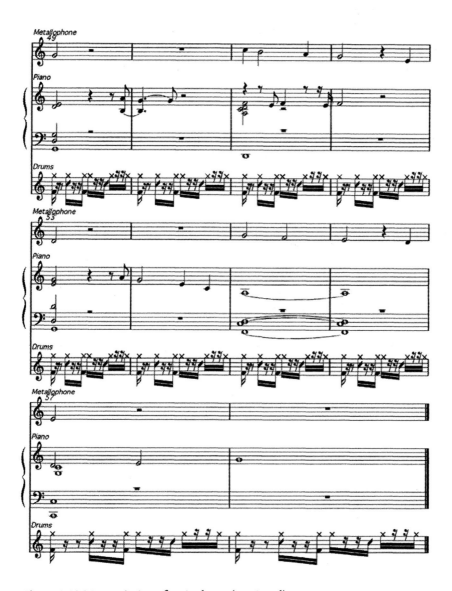

Figure 6.12 Transcription of Episode 12 (continued)

In this episode Mark plays long phrases and is involved in *extended play*. The whole improvisation from which the episode is selected is nine minutes long. The melodic lines Mark plays reach over many bars. An example of these extended melodies can be seen in the transcription of bars 3–10 (Figure 6.13).

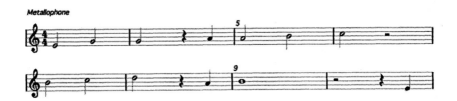

Figure 6.13 Bars 3–10 of Episode 12

The harmonic tempo, or speed with which the music moves from one chord to the next, reflects the two-bar phrasing of Mark's melodic forms. This structure originates from the first two phrases in bars 3–4 and 5–6, and is used throughout the episode. An example of the two-bar harmonic tempo is seen in bars 7–14 (Figure 6.14).

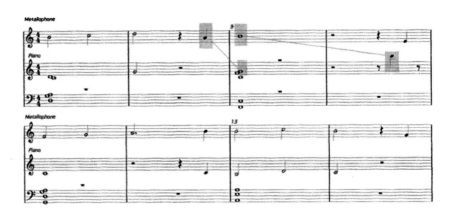

Figure 6.14 Bars 7–14 of Episode 12

The therapist plays new harmony chords at bars 7, 9, 11 and 13. Mark *leads* the direction of the improvisation in two ways. First he leads the melodic contours by beginning the melody phrases on the fourth crotchet of many of the phrases. This is apparent in bars 8, 10, 12 and 14.

Mark also *leads* the therapist in his choice of harmonic accompaniment on the piano. We can see that on the upbeat to bar 9 Mark plays the tone 'a' followed by the tone 'b'. Perhaps the therapist expected Mark to play the tone 'g' at this point, the neighbouring tone to 'a'. This may explain why the F major chord in bar 9 played by the therapist includes the additional ninth interval, the tone 'g'. The therapist releases the harmonic tension created by the tone 'b' played by Mark in bar 9 by sounding the high 'c' on the second half of the third beat in bar 10. This long suspension, of over one-and-a-half bars, is released very shortly before Mark begins the next melodic phrase and adds a sense of forward movement.

Mark and the therapist improvise in this episode in a manner that suggests equality in musical roles. Mark is clearly extemporizing upon a recognizable melodic and temporal unit; the therapist's accompaniment is sparse, but precise, and musically related to the harmonic suggestions made by the contours of Mark's melodies.

Summary of Episodes 9–12 from therapy with Mark

Mark was referred to individual music therapy at a time when he was unable to move. The first episode (Episode 9) is selected from a later point in time, as he was able to move his left hand a few centimetres. At this time Mark and the therapist were challenged to find a way to meet his wish in overcoming these severe constraints of movement. Mark was aware of the restrictions caused by his movement disorders and was interested in trying out ways of overcoming them. With the use of a synthesizer it became possible for Mark to participate in instrumental music making. A speech disorder disturbed Mark in using his vocal chords and he was not comfortable singing. Therefore, instrumental music making offered him the opportunity to participate in rhythmic and melodic movement.

In Episode 9 we see how he is able to create aesthetically pleasing musical gestures. The melodic form of Episode 9 reflects a curve, climaxing at the two-thirds point, and returning to rest at the point of departure. The emotional quality of this improvisation is an indicator of his quiet and reflective mood at the time. He was almost completely unable to move his body without assistance and was heavily reliant on help from others. In this episode Mark was able to be independent in his use of the synthesizer. He was able to literally 'move' from one tone to another and create a gesture of movement in musical form. The device used to control the synthesizer did not allow completely free movement and was limited to playing only a small selection of pitches. Nevertheless, the pop-ballad style of the improvisation reflects the 'contented' atmosphere surrounding Mark and the therapist, who have together found a way to overcome the physical movement restrictions that limit the musical ability of one of the players.

In commenting on this improvisation at the end of his rehabilitation treatment Mark said:

> I could play a melody at all with the reduced movement…with the hand torch and a possibility was opened which I did simply not have before. To play this melody at all, albeit restricted, because I could only play tones next to each other and in a volume level and a particular length, was a step forward, which also made a lot of fun to play, simply getting away from the usual environment practically. (translation from clinical notes)

As Mark regained the ability to partially move his left lower arm he was able to control the synthesizer using a touch-sensitive keyboard. In Episode 10 we see the increase in expression in his playing. Where Episode 9 is in the style of a light pop-ballad, Episode 10 is characterized by a more serene and sorrowful mood. The harmonic vocabulary and dynamic expression used in the improvisation are more complex and sophisticated. Mark commented on this improvisation: 'That is one for me, one from the most beautiful pieces where one gets into dreaming and a piece where one can hear the difference to the first' (from clinical notes). At this stage, Mark is developing his own musical identity. His style of improvisation is recognizable and he extends his musical expression.

At the time from which Episode 11 was selected Mark was experimenting with acoustic instruments. His movement range had expanded and he was able to play using a beater. He had become more intensively involved with his **musical expression** and playing abilities and his **motility**. The improvisations were becoming larger in duration and expressive in range. The therapist had begun to refrain completely from *being directive* and Mark became more independent in his music making. Episode 11 is taken from an improvisation in which the therapist stops playing after approximately five minutes and takes on the role of an active listener during the final three minutes. Mark's comments about the improvisation were:

> By this piece I went fairly near to my limits. That was the first time Simon played more in the background. And whilst playing I didn't even notice that at the end he wasn't playing at all – and that I was alone on the steel drum. That was somehow, what I wanted to know – simply to know, 'How far can I go by playing?' (from clinical notes)

Mark challenged himself and tested his boundaries both physically and mentally. This was a significant step in his rehabilitation process. Initially Mark was challenged by the motor disorders, seeking ways to regain autonomy in active movements. He increasingly became able to move his arms and hands. His legs and torso were more severely affected and he was not able to move these parts actively. Over time he was learning to live with his movement possibilities, and not attempting to confront his movement disorders exclusively. Naturally he was intent on reaching a level of independence that he found acceptable for himself. This is a process of readjusting and becoming accustomed to new possibilities in movement.

During this phase, new patterns of movements become integrated into the habits of everyday life. Adjusting to new habits is of great importance in the rehabilitation processes. Once this foundation is laid it is possible for the individual to re-begin a process of growth and development. If we look at rehabilitation as re-finding an ecological niche, then this new repertoire of movements and expressive forms is central to achieving both communication and identity (Aldridge 2005).

In Episode 11 Mark tests his abilities in using his movement possibilities whilst being creatively active. He is using music as a medium of action in which he can hear and feel his development and growth.

Episode 12 is characterized by the equality of musical roles between the patient and therapist and reflects the process of a reducing physical dependency. An increase in self-dependency and **agency** is apparent in the analysis of the four episodes taken from Mark's therapy. Self-dependency and agency show how Mark strives for a balance of equality within the therapeutic relationship.

This balance has been demonstrated in the analysis of Episode 12. Patient and therapist are interwoven in an improvisation where musical roles are finely attuned. The two players reach a dialogical equilibrium. The musical interaction is seamless and balanced. As we talked about the improvisation Mark said:

> I think that this piece will always remain in my memory because it worked so well. And if I can still remember, I can also recollect with happiness the time right at the beginning how it all developed – from simple tones up to this self-played piece which sounds relatively good – when I think back how I used the micro-switch with my head – that is an enormous development. And I think that in this relationship this is one of the best forms of therapy for me, simply to usurp all the momentary possibilities and to make the best out of it. Then you can recognize in the recordings a bit of development from the first piece with the hand torch to this with the metallophone, and the drum machine in the background. That is really an enormous experience, mostly because I had previously only listened to music and never made music myself. Then something happens to you like this – and one comes to play music yourself – that is really something special. (from clinical notes)

As Aldridge (2005) has suggested, many of the problems of neurological rehabilitation are those of dialogical degeneration. Making music together achieves dialogue; it is an activity predicated on the potential of generation for both participants.

CHAPTER 7

The Narrative Explicated

In this final stage of the analysis we try and piece together what the varying episodes mean to us in terms of the 'case' neurological rehabilitation for people who have had their brains traumatically injured. To do this we need to move to another level of abstraction and identify core categories on which we can build that narrative. These core categories are the concepts that stand for what the 'story' is about. In Kellyian terms these would be superordinate constructs (Kelly 1995). As none of the original categories completely capture the essence of this story, we return to the principal components analysis (see Figure 3.2) and re-analyse the relationships between the categories elicited from the constructs and the episodes. In Figure 7.1 we see that the constructs and episodes are organized in two-dimensional space. The calculation for these spatial locations is made according to the rank-ordering of the constructs that the therapist made. On the diagram itself we see two dotted lines: one vertical, one horizontal. These dotted lines represent the two principal axes on which the constructs and episodes are organized. By understanding what these axes can mean, giving them names, and coupling these with the musical episodes and therapeutic experience, then we can begin to identify the narrative. This is not simply a computer analysis – we need to interpret the result. Indeed, as any statistician will tell us, using a statistical analysis program requires knowledge of the data and its relationship to reality. What the computer makes is only a suggestion; we must know what the data mean.

The process of identifying core categories

The categories **communication, emotionality** and **agency** appear near to the x (horizontal) axis. The categories **musical expression, participation** and **motility** are nearer to the y (vertical) axis. With this in mind, two new superordinate categories for the poles of the two axes have been generated: *isolated–integrated* (x axis) and *idiosyncratic–conventional* (y axis) (see Figure 7.1).

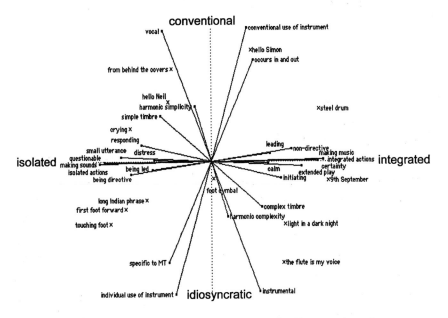

Figure 7.1 The superordinate categories conventional–idiosyncratic and isolated–integrated as polarities of the two main axes

Isolated

The category *isolated* is derived from **communication** (constructs: *small utterance, questionable, making sounds, isolated actions* and *being directive*), **agency** (*being led*) and **emotionality** (*responding* and *distress*).

Being *isolated*, is defined as 'far away from other people, having minimal contact or little contact with others' (Soanes & Stevenson 2003). The term is rooted in the Latin word *insula*, meaning an 'island' (ibid.). We may speak of isolated people as being in isolation. However, becoming isolated is a process and not simply a status, and can be reversed. Isolation refers to a type of contact and not a situation of no contact. Aldridge (1998, 2004b) refers elsewhere to the fact that the process of isolation is critical in the escalation of distress. Our responsibilities as therapist, friends and family are to see how we can reverse that process, even though there are seemingly insurmountable physical and psychological barriers.

Integrated

Being *integrated* derives from **communication** (*non-directive, making music, integrated actions, certainty* and *extended play*), **agency** (*leading* and *initiating*) and **emotionality** (*calm*).

To 'integrate' is to 'combine with another to form a whole, bring into equal participation in or membership of a social group' (Soanes & Stevenson 2003). The word derives from the Latin *integrat*, meaning 'made whole', from *integer*, meaning 'whole' (ibid.). For many years holistic medicine was seen as an ideal. The clinic at Klinik Holthausen, in its initial inception, was based on a holistic perspective and music therapy way seen as a pioneering form of complementary medicine (Aldridge 1988, 1990, 1991). Rather than being seen as a complementary approach, music therapy has become part of the modern medical perspective known as integrative medicine (Aldridge 2001, 2004b).

Idiosyncratic

The category *idiosyncratic* derives from **musical expression** (*harmonic complexity* and *complex timbre*), **participation** (*specific to music therapy*) and **motility** (*individual use of instrument* and *instrumental*).

Idiosyncratic has 'idiosyncrasy' at its root, meaning 'a mode of behaviour or way of thought peculiar to an individual' (Soanes & Stevenson 2003). The term derives from the Greek *idiosunkrasia*, from *idios*, meaning 'own, private', *sun*, meaning 'with', and *krasis*, meaning 'mixture' (ibid.). This is what we find in such clinical situations: complex and private responses that are personal to the patient but inaccessible to any interpretation of meaning by others in the environment. The danger is that this status and the associated isolated movements are interpreted as being reflexive and as having no meaning (see Herkenrath 2002 and in Aldridge 2005). Indeed, some of these movements are reflexive but it is our obligation to convert what is appropriate in these movements, when possible, and bring them into an ecology of meaning.

Conventional

The category *conventional* derives from **musical expression** (*harmonic simplicity* and *simple timbre*), **participation** (*occurs in and out*) and **motility** (*vocal* and *conventional use of instrument*).

Conventional means 'based on or in accordance with what is generally done or believed' (Soanes & Stevenson 2003). The Latin root is *conventio(n)*, meaning 'meeting, covenant' (ibid.). At the centre of the concept is people 'coming together for a meeting or an activity' from *con*, meaning 'together', and *venire*, meaning 'come' (ibid.). And this is what happens in therapy – we bring people together to achieve what is normal. For patients and their families being 'normal' is a central goal. That they can be together again is a primary aim.

Identifying a pattern of change

If we look at the chronological order of the episodes, plotted on the principal components analysis, we can see a clear grouping of Bert in episodes 1–4, Neil in Episodes 5–8 and Mark in Episodes 9–12 (Figure 7.2). The arrowed lines link episodes selected from each of the three patients.

From this perspective, we can see movement of Episodes 1–4 from the bottom left quadrant to the bottom right quadrant. Episode 3 shows that in the process of therapy progressive change takes place in sometimes contrary directions before reaching a new dimension. Episodes 5–8 show movement from the upper left quadrant to the upper right quadrant. Episodes 9–12 move from the lower right quadrant towards the upper right quadrant. Episode 12 returns over the quadrant boundary, but the overall movement from Episode 9 to 12 is upward.

To understand the processes of therapy in the three cases we will need to consider these in context of the pole categories (see Figure 7.2).

For Bert the first three episodes are characterized by *isolated– idiosyncratic* behaviour. The fourth episode shows strong movement towards *idiosyncratic–integrated* behaviour. There is also a reduction in the

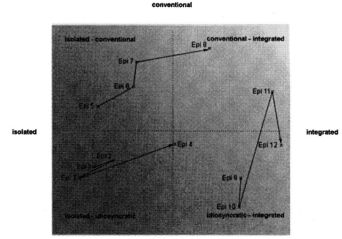

Figure 7.2 Principal components analysis showing the chronological order of the episodes selected from the three cases: Bert (Episodes 1–4), Neil (Episodes 5–8) and Mark (Episodes 9–12)

idiosyncratic nature of the episode, and we can see change on the *idiosyncratic–conventional* axis.

In Neil's music therapy the first three episodes are characterized by *isolated-conventional* behaviour. Showing a continual tendency towards more *conventional* qualities, the final episode clearly demonstrates change in a *conventional–integrated* manner.

Mark's music therapy initially shows change in an increase of *idiosyncratic* nature; the clearest change takes place in the *conventional* nature of the episode. A change towards equality between idiosyncratic and conventional behaviour is seen in the final episode. Nevertheless, the general change is from *idiosyncratic–integrated* behaviour to *conventional–integrated* behaviour.

By viewing the patterns of change demonstrated in terms of the pole categories, we can see that music therapy has facilitated change in all three patients towards *conventional–integrated* behaviour (Figure 7.3).

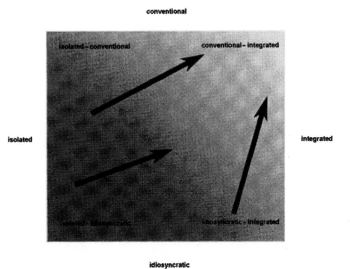

Figure 7.3 A general pattern of change towards conventional–integrated behaviour

Traumatic brain injury is disastrously damaging. Its consequences are sudden, widespread and potentially fatal. Lives are dramatically changed both for the patient and his or her loved ones. In this book we have looked at how music in therapy can be used to rehabilitate people in the early stage of the neurorehabilitation process, who have experienced TBI.

The needs of these individuals are complex, and this study has only considered short episodes in individual creative music therapy in the lives of three people who have experienced TBI. However, these three people are representative of a portfolio of other instances that occurred in the same setting.

What we have found is that people are initially isolated and idiosyncratic in their behaviour. What then happens is that, through the music therapy, by 'catching' those movements and utterances, idiosyncratic behaviours move along the axis of integration towards conventionality. As the process continues these behaviours become more conventional and increasingly integrated with the behaviours from themselves and with others. It may seem strange to people that we emphasize conventionality and integration, when artistic endeavour is often concerned with unconventionality and uniqueness of expression. But the setting changes everything here. We are dealing with the recovery of someone who has been dramatically traumatized and deeply damaged. Returning to a normal life is paramount. Gaining an identity as a normal person is the first and foremost consideration.

The recognition of the importance of reducing of isolation and idiosyncratic behaviour is a significant step towards understanding the patient's needs in neurorehabilitation. Whereas many therapy strategies in neurorehabilitation focus on regaining functional ability, this book shows how music therapy broadens the potential of treatment aspects in neurorehabilitation. Some authors argue that there is an imbalance in the focus of neurorehabilitation towards functional physical ability and emotional and psychosocial aspects of rehabilitation are neglected (Jochims 1992; Magee 1999). This book restores that balance.

People attending neurorehabilitation are not seen in this study from a mechanical or purely medical perspective, but as communicative, expressive and reflective beings. The basis of the approach to music therapy in this study rests on the recognition of the possibilities and abilities of the patient and the value these have in the *performed identity* of each human being (Aldridge 1995). In the study of the improvised performed identity of the three individuals in this study, we have been able to follow the emerging analysis of a collection of significant events as they are interpreted by the therapist. These episodes have been joined or distinguished through constructs eliciting the nature of the phenomena. Correlations between the constructs have led to the identification of categories, terms that hint towards the essence of the processes of change in music therapy.

The three individuals in this study, after setting off from contrasting points, have demonstrated change towards conventional–integrated behaviour over the course of music therapy in early neurorehabilitation. Conventional–integrated behaviour means that those people begin to communicate and are understood by others. No longer isolated and idiosyncratic, they are returned as active human beings within a community of significant others. This is surely the aim of rehabilitation in general, and will remain a significant aspect in later stages of rehabilitation. The development of awareness of the environment and some level of communication, by people who have experienced TBI, in music therapy is described in the literature. Some authors have also highlighted the possibilities music therapy offers for emotional expression and affecting mood state. This present study expands on the literature in suggesting a general pattern of change towards conventional–integrated behaviour, characterized by positive changes in the areas of communication, participation, emotionality, agency, musical expression and motility.

The core narrative category is relationship

In qualitative research, a central feature is to establish a core category that has explanatory value of the significance of the changes in terms of the lives of the individuals. The essence of the categories presented here is their relevance in determining **relationship**.

A relationship refers to 'the way in which two or more people or things are connected' (Soanes & Stevenson 2003), and portrays the *relation* between them. 'Relation' derives from the Latin *relatio(n)*, from *referre*, meaning 'bring back' (ibid.). And this is what happens here. Bert, Neil and Mark are brought back to their lives and families.

In the first stages of developing a relationship with a patient, the music therapist determines the relation between the musical actions and directs the patient's and his or her own attention to the patient's actions. This is necessary to confront the quality of isolation presented by the patient. The idiosyncratic nature of his or her movements or vocalization may be extreme and the therapist will meet the patient's individual repertoire of musical gestures. This is done using synchronization and imitation within a flexible temporal organization. In this way the patient has the opportunity to realize and identify his or her actions and those of others. The therapist also becomes increasingly aware of the patient's abilities and may identify initial attempts towards communication.

Once this is achieved, the therapeutic process is characterized by a phase in which the patient experiences and recognizes the 'link' between his or her actions and those of the therapist. To enhance the conditions the music therapist must be aware of how he or she composes the patient's musical environment. The musical sense of the shared improvisation must be explicit and clear. During this phase there may be a constant recalibration of the amount of directive and non-directive intervention; the therapist may become more certain in his or her interpretation of the patient's actions. This will act as a confirmation of the patient's signs of attributing relation and demonstrate how he or she understands the evolving relationship with the therapist. The patient and therapist are developing a repertoire of relationship-specific communication and will share their own conventions of behaviour. This repertoire of behaviour may contradict or contrast the patient's behaviour observed outside the music therapy setting at this time. This highlights the still somewhat idiosyncratic nature of relating in the music therapy setting.

Later, certainty develops concerning the relation between the patient and the therapist's actions. The therapist reduces the amount of his or her directive interventions. This phase increasingly focuses on the expressive and integrated form of music improvisation. Patient and therapist are able to extend their repertoire of behaviour to include more conventional musical forms, forms that belong to the culture in which they live. Though the music is highly personal, it no longer shows extremes of idiosyncrasy. The music made by the patient is unequivocally his or her own; it belongs to his or her identity. A closeness of partnership in music making emphasizes the essence of the dialogical nature of the therapeutic relationship. The patient has experienced an increase in agency and an interpersonal equality has returned in the life of the patient.

If these steps are achieved we may speak of successful rehabilitation. We 'restore to health or normal life, and former privileges' as a definition of rehabilitation (Soanes & Stevenson 2003). Traumatic brain injury influences an individual's ability to participate in many, if not all, relationships. Having been lost, this participation becomes a privilege. The true work of rehabilitation is to assist people who have experienced TBI to enjoy and develop relationships in their lives. But, more than this, we hope that this book also encourages friends, families and practitioners to try out the other part of the dialogue that is relationship. What is seemingly idiosyncratic and isolated may be a person attempting to communicate. Distress may not simply be a crying out loud but a crying out to. We are that relationship. Our task is to bring them back from the abyss of trauma.

Coda: It's all done by mirrors

We see above that relationship is the core of rehabilitation. Yet we still need to know what the connection is between music and neurological rehabilitation. At the level of social interaction, music events offer possibilities for understanding social and relational events. The process of music making has its ramifications for relating and socializing. Feelings are negotiated in relationship and this is a dynamic, processual activity. Understanding the process of musical improvisation in therapy offers a way of understanding processes in daily life. Understanding the mutuality of music making allows us to understand other social processes of negotiation and relationship. This builds on the premise in Aldridge's earlier works that biological form can be understood through principles of musical form; both are improvised dynamic compositions that occupy a transitory temporal space. Instead of looking at other processes to understand music, we propose that understanding musical process allows us to understand relationship and the dynamics of social forms as per-*form*-ances (Aldridge 2006; Aldridge & Aldridge 2007).

Music is a highly adaptive communication medium that coordinates and manages social interaction (Cross 2006) based upon the temporal regulation of gestural and aural events. Central to the regulation of events for the people that we have read about in this book is the re-establishing of a mutual emotional milieu. Rather than locate emotions in one person, we understand emotions as a description of a pattern of interaction within an ecology of meanings (Aldridge 2000) in a relationship. Meanings are used here as understandings that may not have reached verbal expression. By performing we give expression to the intangible with other people that matter to us. We smile, we talk, we may moan and we can sing. By performing, we move from the isolation of being damaged to the inclusion of being whole regardless of our limitations. To regain the capacities of a functional human being then, make music.

Tia DeNora (2000) has urged us to look at music in everyday life, and she uses music therapy as one of the examples. From her perspective, music not only allows us to feel empowered but is empowering through the gaining of a capacity. We see here in the three studies how capacities are regained and rehabilitated. These capacities are many sided, going further than the functionality of physical movement alone. We do not underestimate the necessity of improving functionality, but to ignore the existential benefits of music making for the people involved here is to neglect a broad spectrum of knowledge about what it is to be human.

Mirror neurons

However, social interaction also has a physical substrate. When we come to investigate what neural mechanisms are involved, then we can only speculate. One avenue of investigation must be that of mirror neurons (Lahav, Saltzman & Schlaug 2007).

From our observations of all three participants, we see and hear that empathy is a central phenomenon of relationship during the early rehabilitation. The therapist reaches out to the patients by matching musical sounds that are based on utterances and gestures that the patient makes.

Gallese, Eagle and Migone (2007) write that the neural circuits activated in a person carrying out actions and expressing emotions are activated through a mirror neuron system in the observer of those actions and emotions. The same neural structures involved in processing and controlling executed actions, felt sensations and emotions are also active when the same actions, sensations and emotions are observed in others (Gallese 2003). We share a common activation of neurons and this commonality is the basis for our inference of the emotional states of the other person with whom we interact (Schulte-Ruther *et al.* 2007). Incidentally, it is a dysfunction in this mirror neuron system that is hypothesized as being the basis of the emotional (Hadjikhani *et al.* 2006) and social deficits in children with autism spectrum disorders (Dapretto *et al.* 2006) that lead to social isolation (Iacoboni & Dapretto 2006). As we have seen, achieving a movement from isolation to integration is the central narrative of this book. We mean movement here both metaphorically and literally. The smallest of bodily movements are captured here, and imitated, in that moving temporal and relational space we call music.

For all three people that we have discussed here, imitation is an important part of the music therapy. Imitation is an important compositional technique in music and immensely relevant in terms of empathy and social behaviour (Bodini, Iacoboni & Lenzi 2004). We also know that overt imitation facilitates motor abilities (Leonard & Tremblay 2007), that the mimicry of facial expressions influences emotional response and understanding (Moody *et al.* 2007) and that imitatory gestural activities are the precursors of language (Arbib 2005). By imitating facial and hand movements we respond to and reflect neural activity. This is the basis of empathy and the mapping of feelings from one person onto another (Leslie, Johnson-Frey & Grafton 2004), which is our common relational ground.

We argue that the performance of musical interaction is the basis of social communication, and this performance is predicated on the presence of mirror neurons in the case of those suffering TBI. This presumes a neural substrate that is activated in the rehabilitation of capacities. We often see what appears to be the reiteration of a developmental cycle in children as they rehabilitate, where previous capacities are recovered. The people that have made music in this book have such a neural substrate. They have moved, laughed, cried, spoken and sung before the traumatic event. Music therapy provides the relational scaffolding for those latent capacities to be revived once more through those actions in time we call music.

Moving from isolation to integration is both a social and a neural activity. Understanding the sensations, emotions and actions of traumatically brain injured people, with apparently limited capabilities immediately following an accident, can be achieved through making music with them. The substrate of this activity appears to be neural, the common medium is musical.

As we read in Chapter 1, the English neurorehabilitation specialist Barbara Wilson describes rehabilitation as a 'two way process' in which professional staff

> work together with the disabled person to achieve the optimum level of physical, social, psychological, and vocational functioning. The ultimate goal of rehabilitation is to enable the person with a disability to function as adequately as possible in his or her most appropriate environment. (1999, p.13)

We would go beyond this and encourage ability beyond disability. Adequate is not enough. Furthermore, we are that environment. This places responsibility on our functioning as much as the patient's. Just as neurodegenerative diseases are described as dialogical degenerative diseases (Aldridge 2006), then we, with the patient, are the dialogue of rehabilitation. Rehabilitation is involved with habitus, our identity is very much embodied, and this embodiment is relational (Aldridge 2004b). We do not live alone, hence our emphasis on relationship. From the Nordoff–Robbins music therapy perspective we search constantly for potentials and it is in the achievement of potentials that healing takes place and we are lifted from our common disability to our mutual realization. We are the contexts for the other's identity. Functionality is mutual.

References

Adams, R. and Victor, M. (1989) *Principles of Neurology*. New York: McGraw-Hill.

Aldridge, D. (1988) 'Holistic research in a hospital setting.' *Holistic Health 18*, 9–10.

Aldridge, D. (1989) 'Music, communication and medicine.' *Journal of the Royal Society of Medicine 82*, 743–746.

Aldridge, D. (1990) 'Pluralism of practice in West Germany.' *Complementary Medical Research 4*, 14–15.

Aldridge, D. (1991) 'Meaning and expression: the pursuit of the aesthetics in research.' *Holistic Medicine 5*, 177–186.

Aldridge, D. (1993) 'The music of the body: music therapy in medical settings.' *Advances 9*, 1, 17–35.

Aldridge, D. (1995) 'Performed identity: the value of the expressive arts in clinical research.' *Journal of Contemporary Health*, Winter, 49–52.

Aldridge, D. (1996) *Music Therapy Research and Practice in Medicine: From Out of the Silence*. London: Jessica Kingsley Publishers.

Aldridge, D. (1998) *Suicide: The Tragedy of Hopelessness*. London: Jessica Kingsley Publishers.

Aldridge, D. (2000) *Spirituality, Healing and Medicine*. London: Jessica Kingsley Publishers.

Aldridge, D. (2001) 'Music therapy and neurological rehabilitation: recognition and the performed body in an ecological niche.' Retrieved January 2003, last updated November 2001, available from www.musictherapyworld.net.

Aldridge, D. (2002) 'Philosophical speculations on two therapeutic applications of breath.' *Subtle Energies and Energy Medicine 12*, 2, 107–124.

Aldridge, D. (2004a) *Case Study Designs in Music Therapy Research*. London: Jessica Kingsley Publishers.

Aldridge, D. (2004b) *The Individual, Health and Integrated Medicine: In Search of Health Care Aesthetic*. London: Jessica Kingsley Publishers.

Aldridge, D. (2005) *Music Therapy in Neurological Rehabilitation: Performing Health*. London: Jessica Kingsley Publishers.

Aldridge, D. (2006) 'Music, Consciousness and Altered States.' In D. Aldridge and J. Fachner (eds) *Music and Altered States*. London: Jessica Kingsley Publishers.

Aldridge, D. and Aldridge, G. (2002) 'Therapeutic narrative analysis: a methodological proposal for the interpretation of music therapy traces.' Retrieved February 2003, last updated January 2003, available from www.musictherapyworld.net.

Aldridge, D. and Aldridge, G. (2007) *Melody in Music Therapy: A Therapeutic Narrative Analysis.* London: Jessica Kingsley Publishers.

Aldridge, D., Gustorff, D. and Hannich, H. J. (1990) 'Where am I? Music therapy applied to coma patients.' *Journal of the Royal Society of Medicine 83*, 6, 345–346.

Ansdell, G. (1995) *Music for Life: Aspects of Creative Music Therapy with Adult Clients.* London: Jessica Kingsley Publishers.

Arbib, M. A. (2005) 'From monkey-like action recognition to human language: an evolutionary framework for neurolinguistics.' *Behavioral and Brain Sciences 28*, 2, 105–124; discussion 125–167.

Baker, F. (2001) 'The effects of live, taped, and no music on people experiencing posttraumatic amnesia.' *Journal of Music Therapy 38*, 3, 170–192.

Baker, F. and Wigram, T. (2004) 'Rehabilitating the uninflected voice: finding climax and cadence.' *Music Therapy Perspectives 22*, 1, 4–10.

Barker, V. L. and Brunk, B. (1991) 'The role of a creative arts group in the treatment of clients with traumatic brain injury.' *Music Therapy Perspectives 9*, 26–31.

Bischof, S. (2001) 'Musiktherapie mit Apallischen Kindern.' In D. Aldridge (ed.) *Kairos V: Musiktherapie mit Kindern.* Berne: Hans Huber.

Bodini, B., Iacoboni, M. and Lenzi, G. L. (2004) 'Acute stroke effects on emotions: an interpretation through the mirror system.' *Current Opinion in Neurology 17*, 1, 55–60.

Bright, R. and Signorelli, R. (1999) 'Improving Quality of Life for Profoundly Brain-impaired Clients: The Role of Music Therapy.' In R. Rebollo Pratt and D. Erdonmez Grocke (eds) *MusicMedicine 3.* Parkville: University of Melbourne.

Bruscia, K. E. (1991) *Defining Music Therapy.* Phoenixville, PA: Barcelona Publishers.

Burke, D. Alexander, K. Baker, F., Baxter, M. *et al.* (2000) 'Rehabilitation of a person with severe traumatic brain injury.' *Brain Injury 14*, 5, 463–471.

Carlisle, B. J. (2000) The effects of music-assisted relaxation therapy on anxiety in brain injury patients.' Unpublished Masters thesis, Michigan State University, Michigan.

Claeys, M. S., Miller, A. C., Dalloul-Rampersad, R. and Kollar, M. (1989) 'The role of music and music therapy in the rehabilitation of traumatically brain injured clients.' *Music Therapy Perspectives 6*, 71–77.

Cohen, N. S. (1992) 'The effect of singing instruction on the speech production of neurologically impaired persons.' *Journal of Music Therapy 29*, 2, 87–102.

Cross, I. (2006) 'Four issues in the study of music in evolution.' *World of Music 48*, 3, 55–63.

Dapretto, M., Davies, M. S., Pfeifer, J. H., Scott, A. A., *et al.* (2006) 'Understanding emotions in others: mirror neuron dysfunction in children with autism spectrum disorders.' *Nature Neuroscience 9*, 1, 28–30.

DeNora, T. (2000) *Music in Everyday Life.* Cambridge: Cambridge University Press.

Dey, I. (1999) *Grounding Grounded Theory.* London: Academic Press.

Emich, I. F. (1980) 'Rehabilitative potentialities and successes of aphasia therapy in children and young people after cerebrotraumatic lesions.' *Rehabilitation 19*, 3, 151–159.

Friedrichsen, G. (1980) *The Shorter Oxford English Dictionary.* Oxford: Oxford University Press.

Gadomski, M. and Jochims, S. (1986) 'Musiktherapie bei schweren Schaedel-Hirn-Traumen [Music therapy for severe craniocerebral trauma].' *Musiktherapeutische-Umschau 7*, 2, 103–110.

Gallese, V. (2003) 'The roots of empathy: the shared manifold hypothesis and the neural basis of intersubjectivity.' *Psychopathology 36*, 4, 171–180.

Gallese, V., Eagle, M. N. and Migone, P. (2007) 'Intentional attunement: mirror neurons and the neural underpinnings of interpersonal relations.' *Journal of the American Psychoanalytic Association 55*, 1, 131–176.

Gervin, A. P. (1991) 'Music therapy compensatory technique utilizing song lyrics during dressing to promote independence in the patient with a brain injury.' *Music Therapy Perspectives 9*, 87–90.

Gilbertson, S. (1999) 'Music Therapy in Neurosurgical Rehabilitation.' In T. Wigram and J. De Backer (eds) *The Application of Music Therapy in Development Disability, Paediatrics and Neurology.* London: Jessica Kingsley Publishers.

Gilbertson, S. (2002) *Light on a Dark Night.* Music Therapy World Information CD ROM IV. Witten: Music Therapy World.

Gilbertson, S. (2005) 'Music Therapy in Neurorehabilitation after Traumatic Brain Injury: A Literature Review.' In D. Aldridge (ed.) *Music Therapy in Neurological Rehabilitation: Performing Health.* London: Jessica Kingsley Publishers.

Glanville, H. J. (1982) 'What is Rehabilitation?' In L. Illis (ed.) *Neurological Rehabilitation.* Oxford: Blackwell Scientific Publications.

Glassman, L. R. (1991) 'Music therapy and bibliotherapy in the rehabilitation of traumatic brain injury: a case study.' *Arts in Psychotherapy 18*, 2, 149–156.

Hadjikhani, N., Joseph, R. M., Snyder, J. and Tager-Flusberg, H. (2006) 'Anatomical differences in the mirror neuron system and social cognition network in autism.' *Cerebral Cortex 16*, 9, 1276–1282.

Herkenrath, A. (2002) 'Musiktherapie und Wahrnehmung: Ein Beitrag der Musiktherapie zur Evalierung der Wahrnehmungsfähigkeit bei Patienten mit schweren Hirnverletzungen.' In D. Aldridge and M. Dembski (eds) *Music Therapy World: Musiktherapie, Diagnostik und Wahrnehmung.* Witten: University Witten/Herdecke.

Higgins, R. (1993) *Approaches to Case-study: A Handbook for Those Entering the Therapeutic Field.* London: Jessica Kingsley Publishers.

Hiller, P. U. (1989) 'Song story: a potent tool for cognitive and affective relearning in head injury.' *Cognitive Rehabilitation 7*, 2, 20–23.

Hohmann, W. (1987) 'Erfahrungen in der Auditiven Musiktherapie mit Hirngeschaedigten [Experiences with auditive music therapy with brain-damaged patients].' *Musiktherapeutische-Umschau 18*, 3, 178–192.

Hurt, C. P., Rice, R. R., McIntosh, G. C. and Thaut, M. H. (1998) 'Rhythmic auditory stimulation in gait training for patients with traumatic brain injury.' *Journal of Music Therapy 35*, 4, 228–241.

Iacoboni, M. and Dapretto, M. (2006) 'The mirror neuron system and the consequences of its dysfunction.' *National Review of Neuroscience 7*, 12, 942–951.

Jochims, S. (1990) 'Coping with illness in the early phase of severe neurologic diseases. A contribution of music therapy to psychological management in selected neurologic disease pictures.' *Psychotherapie, Psychosomatik, Medizinische Psychologie 40*, 3–4, 115–122.

Jochims, S. (1992) 'Emotionale Krankheitsverarbeitungsprozesse in der Fruehphase erworbener zerebraler Laesionen [Emotional processes in coping with disease in the early stages of acquired cerebral lesions].' *Musik-, Tanz- und -Kunsttherapie 3*, 3, 129–136.

Jochims, S. (1994) 'Kontaktaufnahme im Fruehstadium schwerer Schaedel-Hirn-Traumen: Klang als Brucke zum verstummten Menschen.' [Establishing contact in the early stage of severe craniocerebral trauma: sound as the bridge to mute patients.] *Krankengymnastik: Zeitschrift fur Physiotherapeuten 46*, 10, 1316–1324.

Jones, C. P. (1990) 'Spark of life.' *Geriatric Nursing 11*, 4, 194–196.

Jones, R., Hux, K., Morton-Anderson, K. A. and Knepper, L. (1994) 'Auditory stimulation effect on a comatose survivor of traumatic brain injury.' *Archives of Physical Medicine and Rehabilitation 75*, 2, 164–171.

Jungblut, M. (2003) 'Rhythmisch-melodisches Stimmtraining auf musiktherapeutischer Grundlage mit Broca- und Globalaphasikern in der Langzeitrehabilitation.' Unpublished doctoral thesis. Witten: Institute of Music Therapy, University Witten/ Herdecke.

Kelly, G. (1955) *The Psychology of Personal Constructs (vols I and II)*. New York: Norton.

Kennelly, J. and Edwards, J. (1997) 'Providing music therapy to the unconscious child in the paediatric intensive care unit.' *Australian Journal of Music Therapy 8*, 18–29.

Kennelly, J., Hamilton, L. and Cross, J. (2001) 'The interface of music therapy and speech pathology in the rehabilitation of children with acquired brain injury.' *Australian Journal of Music Therapy 12*, 13–20.

Khan, H. I. (1991) *Sufi Teachings. The Art of Being*. Shaftesbury: Element Books.

Kirkpatrick, E. M. (ed.) (1983) *Chambers 20th Century Dictionary*. Edinburgh: Chambers.

Knox, R. and Jutai, J. (1996) 'Music-based rehabilitation of attention following brain injury.' *Canadian Journal of Rehabilitation 9*, 3, 169–181.

Lahav, A., Saltzman, E. and Schlaug, G. (2007) 'Action representation of sound: audiomotor recognition network while listening to newly acquired actions.' *Journal of Neuroscience 27*, 2, 308–314.

Lee, C. (1996) *Music at the Edge: Music Therapy Experiences of a Musician with AIDS*. London: Routledge.

Lee, K. and Baker, F. (1997) 'Towards integrating a holistic rehabilitation system: the implications for music therapy.' *Australian Journal of Music Therapy 8*, 30–37.

Lemkuhl, L. D. (1992) 'The brain injury glossary.' Centre for Neuro Skills. Available from www.neuroskills.com/tbi/hdi/glossary.shtml (accessed on 30/01/08).

Leonard, G. and Tremblay, F. (2007) 'Corticomotor facilitation associated with observation, imagery and imitation of hand actions: a comparative study in young and old adults.' *Experimental Brain Research 177*, 2, 167–175.

Leslie, K. R., Johnson-Frey, S. H. and Grafton, S. T. (2004) 'Functional imaging of face and hand imitation: towards a motor theory of empathy.' *Neuroimage 21*, 2, 601–607.

Livingston, F. (1996) '"Can rock music really be therapy?" Music therapy programs for the rehabilitation of clients with acquired brain injury.' *Australasian Journal of Neuroscience 9*, 1, 12–14.

Lucia, C. M. (1987) 'Toward developing a model of music therapy intervention in the rehabilitation of head trauma patients.' *Music Therapy Perspectives 4*, 34–39.

Magee, W. L. (1999) 'Music therapy within brain injury rehabilitation: to what extent is our clinical practice influenced by the search for outcomes?' *Music Therapy Perspectives 17*, 1, 20–26.

Magee, W. L. and Davidson, J. W. (2002) 'The effect of music therapy on mood states in neurological patients: a pilot study.' *Journal of Music Therapy 39*, 1, 20–29.

Moody, E. J., McIntosh, D. N., Mann, L. J. and Weisser, K. R. (2007) 'More than mere mimicry? The influence of emotion on rapid facial reactions to faces.' *Emotion 7*, 2, 447–457.

Murray, C. and Lopez, A. (1997) 'Global mortality, disability, and the contribution of risk factors: Global Burden of Disease Study.' *Lancet 349*, 1436–1442.

Murray, G. D., Teasdale, G. M., Braakman, R., Cohadon, F., *et al.* (1999) 'The European Brain Injury Consortium Survey of Head Injuries.' *Acta Neurochirurgica 141*, 3, 223–236.

National Institute of Health Consensus Development Panel on Rehabilitation of Persons with Traumatic Brain Injury (1999) 'Rehabilitation of persons with traumatic brain injury.' *Journal of the American Medical Association 282*, 10, 974–983.

Nayak, S., Wheeler, B. L., Shiflett, S. C. and Agostinelli, S. (2000) 'Effect of music therapy on mood and social interaction among individuals with acute traumatic brain injury and stroke.' *Rehabilitation Psychology 45*, 3, 274–283.

Noda, R., Moriya, T., Ebihara, T., Hayashi, N. *et al.* (2003) 'Clinical Evaluation of Musico-kenetic Therapy for Patients with Brain Injury during the Sub-acute Phases.' In M. Shigemori and T. Kanno (eds) *Proceedings of the 12th Annual Meeting of the Society for Treatment of Coma*. Tokyo: Society for Treatment of Coma.

Nordoff, P. and Robbins, C. (1977) *Creative Music Therapy: Individualized Treatment for the Handicapped Child*. New York: John Day Company.

Oyama, A., Arawaka, Y., Oikawa, H., Owada, H. *et al.* (2003) 'Trial of Musicokinetic Therapy for Traumatic Patients with Prolonged Disturbance of Consciousness: Two Case Reports.' In M. Shigemori and T. Kanno (eds) *Proceedings of the 12th Annual Meeting of the Society for Treatment of Coma*. Tokyo: Society for Treatment of Coma.

Paul, S. and Ramsey, D. (2000) 'Music therapy in physical medicine and rehabilitation.' *Australian Occupational Therapy Journal 47*, 3, 111–118.

Price-Lackey, P. and Cashman, J. (1996) 'Jenny's story: reinventing oneself through occupation and narrative configuration.' *American Journal of Occupational Therapy 50*, 4, 306–314.

Purdie, H. (1997) 'Music therapy with adults who have traumatic brain injury and stroke.' *British Journal of Music Therapy 11*, 2, 45–50.

Robb, S. L. (1996) 'Techniques in song writing: restoring emotional and physical well-being in adolescents who have been traumatically injured.' *Music Therapy Perspectives 14*, 1, 30–37.

Robinson, G. (2001) 'An investigation of immediate and short-term influences of music, as a therapeutic medium, on brain-injured patients' communication and social interaction skills.' *British Journal of Occupational Therapy 64*, 6, 304.

Robson, C. (2002) *Real World Research: A Resource for Social Scientists and Practitioner-researchers*. Oxford: Blackwell.

Rosenfeld, J. V. and Dun, B. (1999) 'Music Therapy with Children with Severe Traumatic Brain Injury.' In R. Rebollo Pratt and D. Erdonmez Grocke (eds) *MusicMedicine 3*. Parkville: University of Melbourne.

Schinner, K. M., Chisholm, A. H., Grap, M. J., Siva, P., Hallinan, M. and LaVoice-Hawkins, A. M. (1995) 'Effects of auditory stimuli on intracranial pressure and cerebral perfusion pressure in traumatic brain injury.' *Journal of Neuroscience Nursing 27*, 6, 348–354.

Schmid, W. and Aldridge, D. (2004) 'Active music therapy in the treatment of multiple sclerosis patients: a matched control study.' *Journal of Music Therapy 41*, 3, 225–240.

Schulte-Ruther, M., Markowitsch, H. J., Fink, G. R. and Piefke, M. (2007) 'Mirror neuron and theory of mind mechanisms involved in face-to-face interactions: a functional magnetic resonance imaging approach to empathy.' *Journal of Cognitive Neuroscience 19*, 8, 1354–1372.

Scruton, R. (1999) *The Aesthetics of Music.* Oxford: Oxford University Press.

Soanes, C. and Stevenson, A. (eds) (2003) *Oxford Dictionary of English.* Oxford: Oxford University Press.

Strauss, A. (1987) *Qualitative Analysis for Social Scientists.* Cambridge: Cambridge University Press.

Strauss, A. and Corbin, J. (1998) *Basics of Qualitative Research: Techniques and Procedures for Developing Grounded Theory.* London: Sage Publications.

Synder Smith, S. and Winkler, P. (1990) 'Traumatic Head Injuries.' In D. A. Umphred (ed.) *Neurological Rehabilitation.* St Louis: C.V. Mosby Company.

Tamplin, J. (2000) 'Improvisational music therapy approaches to coma arousal.' *Australian Journal of Music Therapy 11,* 38–51.

Tucek, G., Auer-Pekarsky, A.-M. and Stepansky, R. (2001) '"Altorientalische Musiktherapie" bei Schaedel-Hirn-Trauma [Traditional oriental music therapy for traumatic brain injury patients].' *Musik-, Tanz- und -Kunsttherapie 12,* 1, 1–12.

van Dellen, J. R. and Becker, D. P. (1991) 'Trauma of the Nervous System.' In W. G. Bradley, R. B. Darhoff, G. M. Fenichel and C. D. Marsden (eds) *Neurology in Clinical Practice.* Boston: Butterworth-Heinemann.

von Wedel-Parlow, F. K. and Kutzner, M. (1999) 'Neurologische Fruehrehabilitation.' In P. Frömmelt and H. Grötzbach (eds) *Neuro Rehabilitation.* Berlin: Blackwell Wissenschafts-Verlag.

Welter, F. and Schönle, P. (1997) *Neurologische Rehabilitation.* Stuttgart: Fischer Verlag.

Wheeler, B., Shiflett, S. and Nayak, S. (2003) 'Effects of number of sessions and group or individual music therapy on the mood and behaviour of people who have had strokes or traumatic brain injury.' *Nordic Journal of Music Therapy 12,* 2, 139–151.

Wigram, T., Nygaard Pedersen, I. and Bonde, L. O. (2002) *A Comprehensive Guide to Music Therapy: Theory, Clinical Practice, Research and Training.* London: Jessica Kingsley Publishers.

Wilson, B. A. (1999) *Case Studies in Neuropsychological Rehabilitation.* Oxford: Oxford University Press.

Wit, V., Knox, R., Jutai, J. and Loveszy, R. (1994) 'Music therapy and rehabilitation of attention in brain injury: a pilot study.' *Canadian Journal of Music Therapy 2,* 1, 72–89.

World Health Organization (1969) *Technical Report No. 419, 1.2.1.* Geneva: World Health Organization.

World Health Organization (2002) *The World Health Report.* Geneva: World Health Organization.

World Health Organization (2004) 'World report on road traffic injury prevention.' Retrieved May 2004, last update April 2004, available from www.who.int/violence_injury_prevention/publications/road_traffic/world_report/en/index.html

Yamamoto, K., Osora, M., Noda, R. and Maeda, Y. (2003) 'The Importance of Effective Music Selection for Synchronized Musico-Kenetic Therapy in Patients with Disturbances of Consciousness.' In M. Shigemori and T. Kanno (eds) *Proceedings of the 12th Annual Meeting of the Society for Treatment of Coma.* Tokyo: Society for Treatment of Coma.

Yin, R. K. (1994) *Case Study Research, Design and Methods.* London: Sage Publications.

Subject Index

Author Index

CPSIA information can be obtained at www.ICGtesting.com
Printed in the USA
BVOW031700041211

277565BV00004B/8/P